Multi-Level Abdominoplasty

Principles, Practice & Proven Outcomes

Multi-Level Abdominoplasty

Principles, Practice & Proven Outcomes

Or Friedman, MD., MBA

Dina Recanati School of Medicine, Reichman University, Herzelia, Israel
Gray Faculty of Medical & Health Sciences, Tel Aviv University, Tel Aviv, Israel

World Scientific

NEW JERSEY • LONDON • SINGAPORE • BEIJING • SHANGHAI • HONG KONG • TAIPEI • CHENNAI • TOKYO

Published by

World Scientific Publishing Co. Pte. Ltd.
5 Toh Tuck Link, Singapore 596224
USA office: 27 Warren Street, Suite 401-402, Hackensack, NJ 07601
UK office: 57 Shelton Street, Covent Garden, London WC2H 9HE

British Library Cataloguing-in-Publication Data
A catalogue record for this book is available from the British Library.

MULTI-LEVEL ABDOMINOPLASTY
Principles, Practice & Proven Outcomes

ISBN 978-981-98-1808-2 (hardcover)
ISBN 978-981-98-1809-9 (ebook for institutions)
ISBN 978-981-98-1810-5 (ebook for individuals)

For any available supplementary material, please visit
https://www.worldscientific.com/worldscibooks/10.1142/14445#t=suppl

Dedication

In the memory of Dr. **Amiram Borenstien** — master surgeon, steadfast mentor, and cherished friend.

Your rigor in the operating room, and generosity of spirit shaped my craft and character. Co-authoring *Multi-level Mammaplasty* with you remains one of my proudest collaborations. Carrying your lessons forward in these pages is my way of keeping your voice loud and clear.

And to my family – **Sveta, Eva, Helen, and Dani**.

Your patience during the late nights. Your laughter when I needed perspective, and your unwavering belief in me are the bedrock beneath every chapter.

This book exists because of you all.

Acknowledgment

Professor Arnon Afek, the founding dean and the Prof. Cecil Taitz Academic Chair in the Field of Anatomy at the Dina Recanati School of Medicine, Reichman University. And the director of the Gertner Institute, Sheba Medical Center. For his professional and personal support.

Contents

1

Preface—A Journey through the Evolving Landscape of Abdominoplasty

This book provides a comprehensive guide to the evolution and modern practice of abdominoplasty, culminating in the multi-level abdominoplasty technique—a method specifically designed to address the multifaceted challenges presented by patients seeking comprehensive abdominal rejuvenation.

About This Book

This monograph is intended for plastic surgeons at all levels—from residents and fellows to experienced practitioners—seeking to enhance their understanding and technical execution of modern abdominoplasty. Each chapter builds upon fundamental concepts to present an evidence-based, clinically proven approach to abdominal contouring surgery, with particular emphasis on the multi-level abdominoplasty technique developed through two decades of surgical refinement and careful outcomes analysis.

The field of abdominoplasty, a cornerstone of body contouring surgery, has undergone a remarkable transformation since its inception. Driven by a relentless pursuit of improved outcomes, minimized scarring, and enhanced patient satisfaction, surgeons have embarked on a continuous journey of refinement and innovation. Early abdominoplasty techniques, while groundbreaking for their time, were often associated with significant scarring, a limited ability to address the abdomen's complex three-dimensional nature, and the potential for complications.

How to Navigate This Book

This text is organized to provide a logical progression from fundamental concepts to advanced applications:

- Begin with Chapters 2–3 to establish a solid foundation in the essential anatomy and core principles of modern abdominoplasty.
- Proceed to Chapters 4–6 to understand the comprehensive multi-level abdominoplasty technique and its variations, including patient selection, consultation, and lipoabdominoplasty approaches.
- Focus on Chapters 7–10 for specialized applications and advanced techniques, including management of massive weight loss patients (both from bariatric surgery and newer GLP-1 receptor agonist medications), the innovative "paper corset" technique for postoperative management, complication prevention, and cutting-edge scar optimization.

While readers may be tempted to focus on specific chapters of immediate interest, we encourage a sequential reading for a comprehensive understanding of how each technique builds upon fundamental principles.

Historical Foundations and Evolution

The earliest recorded attempts at abdominal contouring date back to Kelly in 1899, who performed one of the first documented panniculectomies—procedures to remove overhanging abdominal skin and fat [1]. Kelly's work, primarily focused on functional improvement rather than aesthetics, established the foundation for future developments in the field. Thorek followed in 1924 with techniques that expanded upon Kelly's approach, focusing more deliberately on the excision of redundant skin and fat to enhance patient mobility and hygiene [2].

Pitanguy's landmark contribution in 1967 revolutionized the procedure. His introduction of the low transverse abdominal incision with the undermining of the abdominal flap to the costal margins and umbilical transposition became a widely adopted standard [3]. Pitanguy, recognized for his artistic approach to plastic surgery, offered improved aesthetic results compared to earlier methods, though his technique often resulted in extensive scarring and did not fully address the nuances of body contour.

The limitations of these traditional approaches became increasingly apparent as surgeons sought to achieve more natural and harmonious results. Lockwood's high lateral tension abdominoplasty with superficial fascial system suspension, introduced in 1995, marked a significant paradigm shift [4]. A pioneer in body contouring, Lockwood strategically redistributed tension and focused on waistline definition through fascial suspension. His technique offered a more refined approach, mitigating tension on the central abdomen and producing a more aesthetically pleasing silhouette.

Navigating the Trade-offs: Toward a Comprehensive Solution

Despite these advancements, challenges remained, particularly for patients with significant skin laxity, diastasis recti (separation of the abdominal muscles exceeding 2–3 cm), and localized fat deposits (lipodystrophy), often seen in the post-bariatric population. The need for a more comprehensive approach, capable of addressing these complex anatomical issues, became increasingly evident.

Unlike traditional abdominoplasty, the multi-level technique integrates layered closure, comprehensive muscle plication, and individualized tension distribution. It represents a holistic evolution in abdominal contouring, combining meticulous muscle repair, strategic fat removal, and a unique, layered closure system that addresses both vertical and horizontal laxity. This approach not only enhances three-dimensional shaping and waistline definition but also reduces complications linked to high-tension closures. Its adaptability allows for tailored solutions across diverse patient populations, including those with massive weight loss.

While the technique may necessitate more extensive dissection to ensure optimal contouring and even tension distribution, this is a calculated trade-off. Patient-reported outcomes have consistently shown high satisfaction rates, with improvements not only in physical appearance but also in functional capacity and quality of life.

Figure 1.1 shows a multi-level abdominoplasty illustration—this detailed illustration showcases the key steps of the technique, such as muscle plication, lateral tension sutures, and the layered closure system. Additional illustrations in subsequent chapters will further demonstrate the technical execution and expected outcomes.

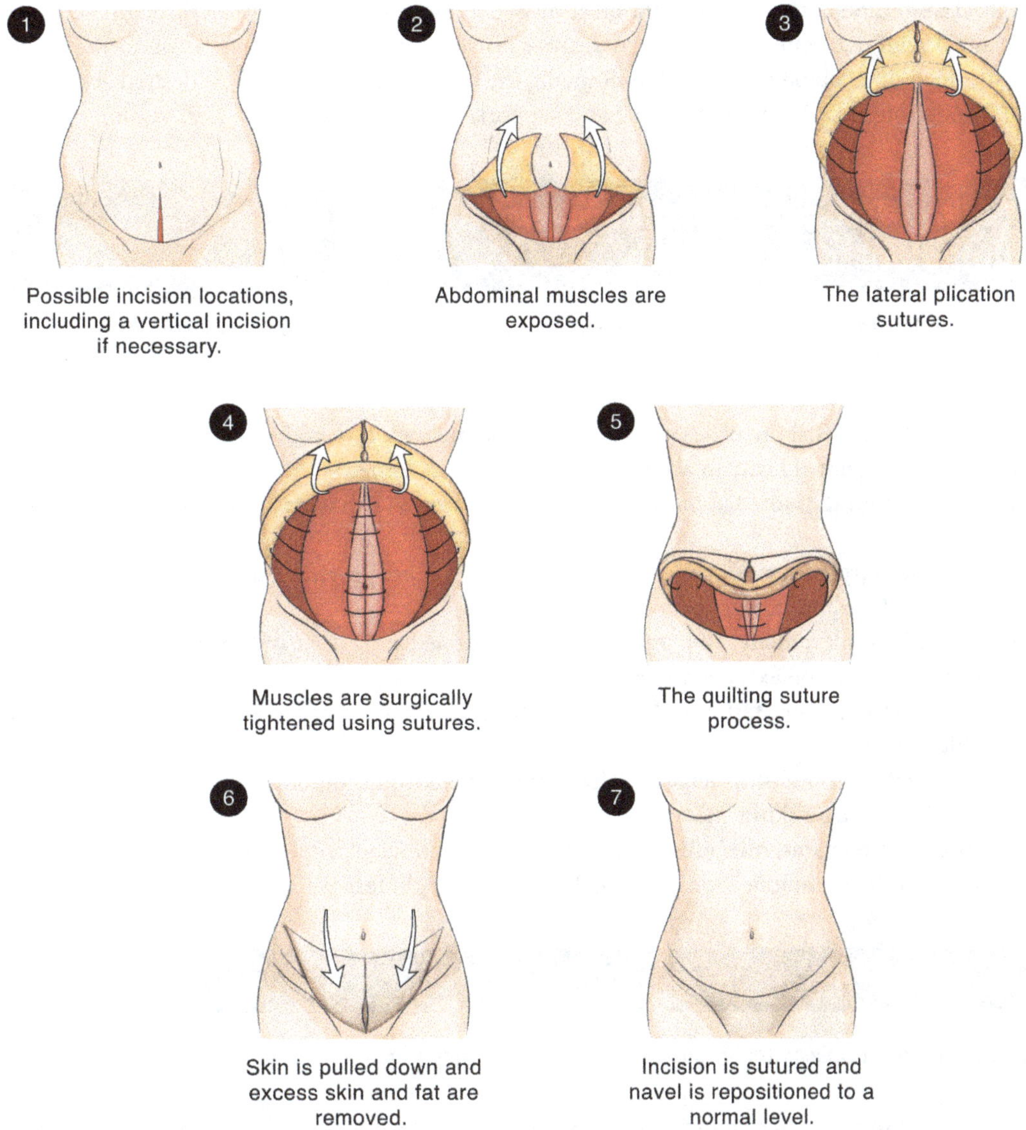

Figure 1.1. ■ **Multi-level abdominoplasty illustration** — This detailed illustration showcases the key steps of the technique, such as muscle plication, lateral tension sutures, and the layered closure system. Additional illustrations in subsequent chapters will further demonstrate the technical execution and expected outcomes.

The Logic of Internal Support: A Paradigm Shift

Central to the multi-level abdominoplasty philosophy is the concept of internal structural support rather than reliance on skin tension for long-term contour maintenance. Traditional techniques often relied heavily on skin tension to achieve the desired shape. However, skin elasticity is a highly variable factor, influenced by age, genetics, weight fluctuations, pregnancies, and other life events.

This reliance presents a precarious dilemma: modest skin tension may minimize tissue necrosis due to ischemia, but often fails to achieve optimal contour. Conversely, higher skin tension may improve the initial aesthetic outcome but significantly increases the risk of necrosis, infection, wound dehiscence (opening), and unsightly, widened scars.

Multi-level abdominoplasty prioritizes the creation of a robust internal framework through meticulous muscle repair and fascial reinforcement, particularly of Scarpa's fascia. The final skin closure is performed with minimal tension, ensuring optimal blood supply and minimizing the risk of complications. The desired abdominal contour is achieved through strategic internal reshaping and support, not through excessive skin tension.

The Guiding Principles of Multi-Level Abdominoplasty: A Commitment to Excellence

The multi-level abdominoplasty technique is guided by a set of core principles that underpin its safety, efficacy, and long-term results:

1. **Addressing both dimensions of laxity**: The technique meticulously addresses both vertical and horizontal components of abdominal laxity to achieve a harmonious outcome.
2. **Building a solid foundation**: Meticulous rectus muscle plication and deep fascial support ensure a strong and durable result.
3. **Comprehensive support system**: The multi-level closure system provides consistent support throughout the abdominal wall, distributing tension evenly.
4. **Strategic umbilical placement**: The umbilicus is repositioned at 61–67% of the xiphoid-pubic distance, with careful attention to natural axis alignment.
5. **Dynamic assessment over static markings**: Real-time adjustments are made during surgery, ensuring the best possible outcome.
6. **Internal support, minimal skin tension**: The goal is a beautifully contoured abdomen supported internally, with minimal reliance on skin tension.
7. **Maximizing improvement, minimizing risk**: The aim is significant improvement in three-dimensional contour while minimizing complications, especially for post-weight loss patients.

Multi-Level Technique Advantages

The multi-level abdominoplasty technique offers several distinct advantages over traditional approaches:

- **Comprehensive muscle plication** from the xiphoid to the pubis with strategic reinforcement provides maximal correction of diastasis recti [7].
- **Lateral tension sutures** create enhanced waistline definition by strategically converting horizontal tissue excess into central support, effectively narrowing the waist while maintaining a natural-appearing contour.
- **Tension distribution** via a layered closure system minimizes wound complications by reducing stress on the incision line [8].
- **Perforator preservation** techniques enhance flap viability and reduce necrosis risk even with extensive dissection [9].
- **Strategic management of Scarpa's fascia** decreases dead space and seroma formation while preserving lymphatic drainage.
- **Tension-free skin closure** promotes optimal scarring patterns and minimizes the risk of wound dehiscence.
- **Adaptability for various patient populations**, including traditional aesthetic patients and the growing demographic of massive weight loss patients, whether from bariatric surgery or newer GLP-1 receptor agonist medications.

These advantages create a comprehensive approach that addresses both aesthetic concerns and functional improvements, with reduced complication rates compared to traditional techniques.

Emerging Patient Populations

A notable development in the field of abdominoplasty is the increasing number of patients seeking body contouring following weight loss achieved through GLP-1 receptor agonist medications (such as semaglutide and tirzepatide). As detailed in Chapter 7, these patients present with unique characteristics that differ from traditional post-bariatric surgery patients, including different patterns of skin laxity, nutritional status, and perioperative management requirements. The multi-level abdominoplasty technique has proven highly adaptable to this emerging patient population, offering excellent aesthetic outcomes while addressing their specific needs.

A Legacy of Innovation: Advancing the Art of Body Contouring

The multi-level abdominoplasty technique offers evidence-based advantages over conventional approaches. Clinical studies have demonstrated reduced seroma formation, improved scar quality, and enhanced long-term contour maintenance compared to traditional techniques. The comprehensive approach to fascial reinforcement has proven particularly beneficial for patients with significant musculofascial laxity.

By addressing the inherent limitations of previous methods and focusing on a comprehensive, anatomically sound approach, this technique offers a safe, effective, and potentially longer-lasting solution for patients seeking abdominal rejuvenation. Its advantages far outweigh the slightly more extensive dissection required. Particularly for those who have undergone massive weight loss, this technique provides a path toward restoring not only their physical form but also their confidence and self-esteem.

Advanced Postoperative Management

This book introduces two significant innovations in postoperative management that complement the multi-level abdominoplasty technique:

1. **The "paper corset" technique** (Chapter 8): This novel approach to postoperative support uses a specialized paper tape application that creates a customized compression garment directly on the patient's skin. This technique provides strategic support to the healing tissues, distributes tension evenly across the abdomen, and has been shown to significantly reduce wound healing complications when maintained for 21 days.
2. **Advanced scar treatments** (Chapter 10): Building on the excellent foundation established by the multi-level technique, this chapter details cutting-edge approaches to scar management, including early laser intervention protocols, energy-based drug delivery systems, and comprehensive management strategies tailored to different patient populations and skin types.

Book Structure and Organization

The following chapters present a logical progression from fundamental concepts to advanced applications:

- Chapters 2–3 cover essential anatomy and core principles.
- Chapters 4–6 detail the multi-level abdominoplasty technique and its variations.
- Chapters 7–10 address special considerations, including massive weight loss patients, postoperative management, complication prevention, and scar optimization.

Each chapter includes clinical pearls, evidence-based recommendations, and practical guidance to help readers implement these techniques successfully in their own practice.

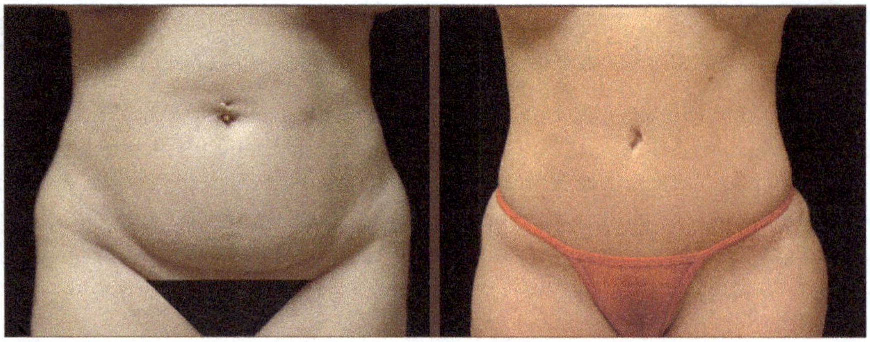

Figure 1.2. ■ **Outcome of multi-level abdominoplasty.** (Left) Pre-operative frontal view displaying combined vertical and horizontal laxity, lower-abdominal adiposity, and attenuated rectus fascia. (Right) Twelve-month post-operative result following multi-level abdominoplasty with full-length rectus plication, lateral-tension fascial suspension, and layered Scarpa-fascial closure. The abdomen is flattened and cinched, the waistline is re-defined, and the low transverse scar lies inconspicuously beneath standard underwear—illustrating the chapter's principle that durable contour is achieved through robust internal support rather than excessive skin tension.

As we look to the future of body contouring, the principles outlined in this text will continue to evolve, driven by ongoing innovation, technological advancements, and a deeper understanding of tissue dynamics. The following chapters will delve into the intricacies of this technique, offering a detailed guide for surgeons seeking to master this advanced approach to abdominal contouring.

References

1. Kelly HA. Report of gynaecological cases. *Johns Hopkins Hospital Bulletin.* 1899; **10**: 197.
2. Thorek M. *Plastic Reconstruction of the Female Breast and Abdomen Wall.* Springfield, IL: Charles C Thomas; 1924.
3. Pitanguy I. Abdominal lipectomy: An approach to it through an analysis of 300 consecutive cases. *Plast Reconstr Surg.* 1967; **40**(4): 384–391. doi:10.1097/00006534-196710000-00001
4. Lockwood T. High-lateral-tension abdominoplasty with superficial fascial system suspension. *Plast Reconstr Surg.* 1995; **96**(3): 603–615. doi:10.1097/00006534-199509000-00010
5. Matarasso A, Swift RW, Rankin M. Abdominoplasty and abdominal contour surgery: A national plastic surgery survey. *Plast Reconstr Surg.* 2006; **117**(6): 1797–1808. doi:10.1097/01.prs.0000218974.36586.2d
6. Brauman D, Capocci J. Liposuction Abdominoplasty: An advanced body contouring technique. *Plast Reconstr Surg.* 2018; **141**(2): 369–379. doi:10.1097/PRS.0000000000004121
7. Saldanha OR, De Souza Pinto EB, Mattos WN Jr, *et al.* Lipoabdominoplasty with selective and safe undermining. *Aesthetic Plast Surg.* 2003; **27**(4): 322–327. doi:10.1007/s00266-003-3027-5
8. Rohrich RJ, Gosman AA, Conrad MH, Coleman J. Simplifying circumferential body contouring: The central body lift evolution. *Plast Reconstr Surg.* 2006; **118**(2): 525–535. doi:10.1097/01.prs.0000227674.14624.24
9. Nahas FX, Ferreira LM, Ghelfond C. Does quilting suture prevent seroma in abdominoplasty? *Plast Reconstr Surg.* 2007; **119**(3): 1060–1064. doi:10.1097/01.prs.0000256488.01465.74
10. Michaels J 5th, Coon D, Rubin JP. Complications in postbariatric body contouring: Postoperative management and treatment. *Plast Reconstr Surg.* 2011; **127**(4): 1693–1700. doi:10.1097/PRS.0b013e318208d1b9
11. Hurvitz KA, Olaya WA, Nguyen A, Wells JH. Evidence-based medicine: Abdominoplasty. *Plast Reconstr Surg.* 2014; **133**(5): 1214–1221. doi:10.1097/PRS.0000000000000347
12. van Uchelen JH, Kon M, Werker PM. The long-term durability of plication of the anterior rectus sheath assessed by ultrasonography. *Plast Reconstr Surg.* 2001; **107**(6): 1578–1584. doi:10.1097/00006534-200105000-00048
13. Batac J, Hamade M, Hamade H, *et al.* Nutritional optimization for postbariatric body contouring: A 10-year experience. *Obes Surg.* 2019; **29**(12): 3962–3970. doi:10.1007/s11695-019-04079-w
14. Gust MJ, Smetona J, Persing JA, *et al.* The impact of rectus plication techniques on abdominal wall mechanics. *Plast Reconstr Surg Glob Open.* 2020; **8**(9): e3126. doi:10.1097/GOX.0000000000003126
15. Swanson E. Prospective outcome study of 360 patients undergoing multi-level abdominoplasty. *Ann Surg.*2022; **277**(5): e1029–e1037. doi:10.1097/SLA.0000000000005401
16. International Society of Aesthetic Plastic Surgery (ISAPS). ISAPS International survey on aesthetic/cosmetic procedures 2022. https://www.isaps.org/discover/about-isaps/global-statistics/

2

Surgical Anatomy of the Abdomen for Abdominoplasty

Introduction

The abdomen, a central component of the human form, is a region of complex anatomical interplay, responsible for vital physiological functions and contributing significantly to aesthetic appearance. For plastic surgeons undertaking abdominoplasty, a nuanced and thorough understanding of abdominal anatomy is not merely beneficial but absolutely paramount to achieving superior aesthetic outcomes, ensuring functional integrity, and minimizing complications. This chapter delves into the intricacies of abdominal anatomy, meticulously examining the relevant structures, their interrelationships, and their profound significance in the context of abdominoplasty. With ongoing advances in surgical techniques, including lipoabdominoplasty and high-definition contouring, this anatomical knowledge becomes increasingly crucial for optimal patient outcomes.

Key Points

- Thorough knowledge of abdominal wall anatomy is fundamental to successful abdominoplasty.
- Understanding of vascular networks helps prevent ischemic complications.
- Recognition of fascial planes influences tissue handling and surgical outcomes.
- Appreciation of nervous and lymphatic systems guides prevention of sensory and edema issues.

Abdominal Boundaries and Surface Anatomy: A Topographical Overview

The abdomen's topographical boundaries are traditionally defined as extending from the inferior margins of the costal arches superiorly to the inguinal ligaments and pubic symphysis inferiorly, with the anterior axillary lines demarcating the lateral extents. Precise identification of surface landmarks is the cornerstone of surgical planning and execution in abdominoplasty. These include:

1. **Xiphoid process**: The cartilaginous, lowermost segment of the sternum, palpable at the superior midline, serves as a crucial reference point for determining the extent of dissection and the superior limit of the linea alba.

2. **Costal margins**: Formed by the inferior borders of the 7th to 10th ribs and the cartilages of the 11th and 12th ribs, these margins dictate the superior extent of the abdominal wall and influence incision placement in certain abdominoplasty techniques.
3. **Anterior superior iliac spines (ASIS)**: Prominent bony projections of the iliac crests, palpable anterolaterally, these are vital landmarks for assessing abdominal wall laxity, determining the lower limits of dissection, and planning the placement of low transverse incisions.
4. **Pubic symphysis**: The cartilaginous joint uniting the left and right pubic bones in the midline, this landmark defines the inferior border of the abdomen and serves as a reference for lower abdominal incisions and muscle plication.
5. **Umbilicus**: A central focal point of the abdomen, typically situated at the level of the L3–L4 intervertebral disc, the umbilicus's position, shape, and relationship to surrounding structures are of paramount aesthetic importance in abdominoplasty.
6. **Inguinal ligaments**: These ligaments run from the ASIS to the pubic tubercle and form the lower boundary of the abdominal wall, serving as important landmarks during lower abdominal dissection.

Clinical pearl: Landmark palpation

When marking the patient preoperatively, have them perform a partial sit-up to facilitate identification of the rectus muscles and any diastasis. The umbilicus position relative to the ASIS helps determine the degree of vertical skin excess, with a lower umbilicus often indicating greater skin laxity requiring more aggressive resection.

The Layered Architecture of the Abdominal Wall: A Stratified Dissection

The abdominal wall is a multilayered structure, a sophisticated composite of tissues, each possessing unique characteristics and surgical significance in abdominoplasty:

Skin

The outermost layer, abdominal skin, displays significant variability in thickness, elasticity, and adherence to underlying tissues. Factors such as age, genetic predisposition, history of pregnancy, weight fluctuations, and sun exposure contribute to this variability. Generally, the skin is thicker in the upper abdomen and gradually thins toward the pubic region. Understanding these variations is crucial when designing and elevating abdominal flaps, anticipating flap viability, and planning scar placement. Stretch marks (striae distensae), often present after pregnancy or significant weight loss, represent areas of dermal thinning and are crucial to consider during surgical planning, as they may influence flap elasticity and healing potential.

The biomechanical properties of abdominal skin directly impact flap advancement and tension distribution. Langer's lines, which reflect the predominant orientation of dermal collagen fibers, run transversely in the upper abdomen and more obliquely in the lower abdomen. Incisions planned parallel to these lines generally heal with less conspicuous scarring, informing the preferred transverse orientation of the lower abdominoplasty incision.

Clinical pearl: Skin assessment

Test skin elasticity by the "pinch test"—poor snap-back after pinching suggests decreased elasticity and potential for excess skin after liposuction. Areas with dense striae have compromised dermal integrity and often exhibit poor elasticity, requiring more aggressive excision rather than relying on skin retraction.

Subcutaneous tissue

This layer, deep to the skin, comprises two distinct strata with differing characteristics:

- **Superficial fatty layer (Camper's fascia)**: This layer is composed of lobules of adipose tissue, interspersed with fibrous septa, and its thickness varies considerably among individuals, influenced by genetics, diet, and overall body composition. This layer is a primary target for liposuction when combined with abdominoplasty, allowing for sculpting and contour refinement.
- **Membranous layer (Scarpa's fascia)**: A deeper, more fibrous layer, continuous with Colles' fascia in the perineum and the superficial fascia of the thigh. Preservation of Scarpa's fascia, particularly in the lower abdomen, is advocated by many surgeons as it may help to maintain lymphatic integrity, potentially reducing the incidence of postoperative seromas and promoting faster resolution of edema [1]. The prospective randomized controlled trial by Costa-Ferreira and colleagues demonstrated that Scarpa-sparing techniques can reduce seroma rates from 9% to as low as 2% [1]. Di Martino and colleagues confirmed these findings using ultrasound evaluation [2]. Scarpa's fascia also provides a stronger layer for anchoring sutures, improving the durability of the repair. Modern approaches to Scarpa's preservation include selective hydro-lipo-dissection techniques described by Brauman and colleagues, which maintain this important fascial layer while allowing complete flap mobilization [3].

Table 2.1: Fascial Layers and Surgical Implications [1, 2]

Fascial Layer	Anatomic Location	Composition	Surgical Consideration
Camper's fascia	Superficial fatty layer	Lobulated adipose with fibrous septa	Primary target for liposuction
Scarpa's fascia	Deep membranous layer	Dense fibrous network	Preservation reduces seroma, improves lymphatic drainage
Deep fascia	Investing fascia over muscles	Fibrous sheet	Important for muscle plication and hernia repair
Transversalis fascia	Deep to transversus abdominis	Continuous fascial plane	Critical boundary for hernia identification

Deep fascia

A thin, yet strong, layer of connective tissue that intimately invests the underlying abdominal muscles. It provides an additional layer of support and is continuous with the thoracolumbar fascia posteriorly, the fascia of the thorax superiorly, and the fascia lata of the thigh inferiorly. While it has a minor role in standard abdominoplasty surgery, it is important when dealing with the closure of hernia repairs or when significant muscle reinforcement is required.

Clinical pearl: Fascial identification

Scarpa's fascia appears as a discrete, whitish fibrous layer during dissection, typically encountered 1–2 cm deep to the dermis. Preservation of this layer in the lower abdomen creates a distinct plane for suturing during closure and, when approximated to the superficial fascial system superiorly, can significantly enhance support and reduce dead space.

Muscular layer: The pillars of abdominal strength and contour

The muscular component of the anterior abdominal wall is a symphony of four paired muscles, each contributing to abdominal wall integrity and aesthetic form:

- **Rectus abdominis**: These paired, strap-like muscles, extending vertically from the costal cartilages (ribs 5–7) and xiphoid process to the pubic crest and symphysis, are the primary focus of muscle plication in abdominoplasty. Their tone and separation (diastasis recti) significantly influence abdominal contour. During pregnancy or with significant weight gain, these muscles can separate along the linea alba, creating a condition known as diastasis recti. Patterns of diastasis include supraumbilical, infraumbilical, complete, and asymmetric presentations, each requiring specific approaches to plication.
- **External oblique**: The most superficial of the lateral abdominal muscles, its fibers course inferomedially (like placing hands in pockets), contributing to trunk flexion, rotation, and lateral bending. Their aponeuroses contribute to the anterior rectus sheath and play a role in defining the lateral abdominal contour.
- **Internal oblique**: Situated deep to the external oblique, the fibers of this muscle run superomedially (perpendicular to the external oblique), contributing to trunk flexion, rotation, and lateral bending. Their aponeuroses contribute to both the anterior and posterior rectus sheaths, forming part of the complex fascial network supporting the abdominal wall.
- **Transversus abdominis**: The deepest of the abdominal muscles, its fibers run transversely, acting like a natural corset, providing core stability and contributing to forced expiration. Its aponeurosis contributes primarily to the posterior rectus sheath. This muscle is increasingly recognized for its importance in core stability and postural control.

The aponeuroses of these lateral muscles intricately interweave to form the rectus sheath, a strong fascial envelope encasing the rectus abdominis muscles. The arrangement of these aponeuroses varies above and below the arcuate line (located approximately midway between the umbilicus and pubic symphysis). Above the arcuate line, the rectus sheath has distinct anterior and posterior layers. Below the arcuate line, all aponeurotic layers pass anterior to the rectus muscle, leaving only the transversalis fascia posteriorly. This anatomical arrangement has important implications for the strength and integrity of muscle plication performed during abdominoplasty.

Clinical pearl: Muscle plication strategy

The anatomical configuration of the rectus sheath means that plication below the arcuate line relies primarily on the anterior sheath for strength. Consider using permanent or long-lasting absorbable sutures in this region, and when repairing significant diastasis, employ a two-layer plication technique to enhance durability. Assessment of muscle tone through palpation during preoperative planning helps determine the aggressiveness of plication needed.

Transversalis fascia

A thin, continuous fascial layer that lines the entire abdominal cavity, lying deep to the transversus abdominis muscle. It represents the final fascial layer before encountering the extraperitoneal fat and peritoneum. It is strengthened in some areas to form ligaments, such as the medial and lateral umbilical ligaments. The transversalis fascia provides an additional layer of support for the abdominal wall and can be incorporated into deeper plication techniques when necessary.

Peritoneum

The innermost serous membrane lining the abdominal cavity, the peritoneum envelops the visceral organs and secretes a small amount of fluid, facilitating smooth organ movement. It is generally not directly involved in standard abdominoplasty procedures but may be encountered during hernia repair or in cases requiring extensive dissection. Inadvertent entry into the peritoneal cavity should be recognized and managed appropriately to prevent complications.

Clinical implication

If peritoneal entry occurs during abdominoplasty, close with a simple running 3-0 or 4-0 absorbable suture. Document the location and size of the defect, and monitor postoperatively for any signs of peritonitis or intestinal herniation.

Key Anatomical Structures: Cornerstones of Abdominoplasty

Certain anatomical structures warrant special attention due to their profound relevance to abdominoplasty:

Linea alba: The midline raphe

A strong, fibrous band extending vertically in the midline from the xiphoid process to the pubic symphysis, the linea alba is formed by the fusion of the aponeuroses of the lateral abdominal muscles. It separates the paired rectus abdominis muscles and is a crucial landmark for muscle plication. Weakening or stretching of the linea alba, often seen in diastasis recti, leads to a midline bulge and loss of abdominal contour. The width of the linea alba varies among individuals and can range from 1–3 cm above the umbilicus to 0.5–2 cm below it, with significant widening possible in patients with diastasis recti [4].

Modern plication techniques focus on recreating appropriate tension along the linea alba, with attention to biomechanical forces. A systematic review by Nahas (Level III evidence) has demonstrated that double-layer plication techniques provide greater long-term durability than single-layer approaches, particularly in cases of severe diastasis [19]. A biomechanical study by van Uchelen and colleagues (Level II evidence) further supports this finding with the measurement of tensile forces and tissue integrity after various plication techniques [5].

Clinical pearl: Plication assessment

The degree of diastasis should be measured at multiple levels: 3 cm above the umbilicus, at the umbilicus, and 3 cm below the umbilicus. A separation greater than 3 cm generally requires plication, but the decision should also consider functional symptoms and aesthetic goals. Mark the lateral borders of both rectus muscles before beginning plication to ensure symmetric repair.

Linea semilunaris: The lateral rectus border

These paired, crescent-shaped tendinous intersections mark the lateral borders of the rectus abdominis muscles. They are formed by the fusion of the aponeuroses of the external oblique, internal oblique, and transversus abdominis muscles. They can be accentuated in very muscular patients and can be a landmark when performing liposuction. The linea semilunaris is also a potential site for Spigelian hernias, which should be assessed during preoperative evaluation.

In high-definition lipoabdominoplasty techniques, the linea semilunaris serves as an important landmark for creating a natural-appearing lateral definition of the rectus muscle.

Umbilicus: The aesthetic centerpiece

The umbilicus, a remnant of fetal circulation, is a critical aesthetic landmark in abdominoplasty. Its position, shape, and contour contribute significantly to the overall abdominal appearance. It is attached to the linea alba by a fibrous stalk containing the remnants of the umbilical vessels (urachus and umbilical arteries). Its blood supply is derived from delicate perforating branches, primarily from the deep inferior epigastric vessels.

Meticulous handling of the umbilicus during abdominoplasty, including careful dissection, preservation of its vascular supply, and skillful re-inset, is essential for achieving natural-looking results. The ideal umbilicus is typically ovoid or slightly vertically oriented, with a slight superior hood and a natural depth. Multiple techniques for umbilical transposition have been described, including the "Mercedes" incision, the "Y-V" advancement, and deepithelialized skin flaps [6].

Studies by Castillo and colleagues have demonstrated that using deepithelialized skin flaps for umbilical reinsertion can create a natural-appearing umbilicus with well-concealed scars [7]. This technique involves creating flaps on the abdominal skin to which the umbilicus is sutured, creating a natural depression and maintaining appropriate projection.

Clinical implication: Umbilical vascular supply

The umbilical stalk typically receives blood supply from small perforators originating from the deep inferior epigastric vessels. Excessive skeletonization of the stalk during abdominoplasty can compromise this delicate vascularity, potentially leading to umbilical necrosis. Maintain at least 1.5–2 cm of tissue around the stalk during dissection, and consider using umbilical "parachuting" techniques that minimize manipulation of the stalk itself.

Tendinous intersections

These are fibrous bands that intersect the rectus abdominis muscle transversely, giving it the characteristic "six-pack" appearance in well-defined individuals. They are typically located at the level of the xiphoid process, the umbilicus, and midway between these two points. They are firmly attached to the anterior rectus sheath but not the posterior sheath. Understanding their presence and location can help in planning liposuction and muscle contouring during abdominoplasty.

In high-definition techniques, these intersections serve as guides for selective liposuction to enhance the athletic appearance of the abdomen. Careful preservation of the fat superficial to these intersections during liposuction can accentuate the natural segmentation of the rectus abdominis.

Vascular Supply: Ensuring Flap Viability

A comprehensive understanding of the abdominal wall's vascular supply is of paramount importance for ensuring flap viability, minimizing complications, and optimizing wound healing in abdominoplasty. The intricate vascular network can be broadly categorized into superficial and deep systems:

Table 2.2: Vascular Territories of the Abdominal Wall [8, 13]

Vascular Zone	Primary Arterial Supply	Clinical Relevance	Risk in Abdominoplasty
Huger Zone I (Central)	Deep epigastric system	Midline flap viability	High risk if extensive undermining
Huger Zone II (Lateral)	Intercostal, subcostal, lumbar perforators	Lateral flap perfusion	Moderate risk, improved with limited dissection
Huger Zone III (Lower)	Superficial epigastric, superficial circumflex iliac, superficial external pudendal	Lower abdominal closure	High risk, vessels often sacrificed

Superficial system: Nourishing the skin and subcutaneous tissues

- **Superficial epigastric vessels**: Arising from the femoral artery and vein, these vessels ascend toward the umbilicus, supplying the skin and subcutaneous tissues of the lower abdomen. They are often sacrificed during abdominoplasty when creating the lower abdominal incision.
- **Superficial circumflex iliac vessels**: Also originating from the femoral vessels, these vessels course laterally, supplying the lower lateral abdominal wall and the region overlying the iliac crest. They may be preserved in limited abdominoplasty techniques but are usually divided in full abdominoplasty.
- **Superficial external pudendal vessels**: These vessels, branching from the femoral vessels, contribute to the vascular supply of the lower central abdomen, mons pubis, and external genitalia. Preservation of these vessels, when possible, can help maintain adequate perfusion to the central lower abdominal tissues.

Deep system: The dominant supply to muscles and overlying tissues

- **Deep inferior epigastric vessels**: These vessels, originating from the external iliac artery and vein just superior to the inguinal ligament, are the dominant vascular supply to the rectus abdominis muscles and the overlying tissues. They ascend within the rectus sheath, initially posterior to the rectus muscle, and give off numerous perforating branches that pierce the muscle and anterior rectus sheath to supply the overlying skin and subcutaneous tissues. These perforators are crucial for flap viability in abdominoplasty and are organized in medial and lateral rows [9].

Rozen and colleagues' detailed studies have demonstrated significant variability in the course and distribution of DIEA perforators, emphasizing the importance of understanding these variations for safe surgical planning [9]. The DIEA typically divides into medial and lateral branches, with the lateral branch typically being dominant in 80% of cases [10].

- **Superior epigastric vessels**: These vessels are the terminal branches of the internal thoracic (mammary) artery and vein. They enter the superior aspect of the rectus sheath and anastomose with the deep inferior epigastric vessels, creating a vital collateral pathway. They primarily supply the upper abdominal wall and become increasingly important for flap viability after the division of the deep inferior epigastric vessels during abdominoplasty.
- **Intercostal and subcostal vessels**: These vessels, arising from the aorta, course along the inferior borders of the ribs and contribute to the blood supply of the lateral abdominal wall and the intercostal muscles. They anastomose with both the superior and inferior epigastric systems, providing additional collateral circulation.

- **Lumbar arteries**: These paired vessels arise from the aorta and supply the posterior abdominal wall, also contributing to the collateral circulation. They become particularly important in ensuring adequate perfusion following extensive undermining of the abdominal flap.

Clinical pearl: Perforator preservation

When performing lipoabdominoplasty, consider preserving large perforating vessels, particularly in the periumbilical region. These can be identified during initial liposuction as areas of increased resistance or bleeding. In massive weight loss patients, where tissue quality may already be compromised, maintaining these key perforators becomes even more critical for flap viability.

The superficial and deep systems form rich and extensive anastomoses, creating a robust vascular network. The **choke vessels** between these systems are crucial for flap survival. These vessels, as described by Taylor and Palmer, represent the narrowed anastomotic connections between adjacent vascular territories [11]. Following surgical interventions that divide primary vessels, these choke vessels can dilate over 48–72 hours, improving circulation to potentially compromised tissues. This concept is particularly important in abdominoplasty, where the deep inferior epigastric vessels are often divided.

Recent angiographic studies have demonstrated that previous abdominal surgery can significantly alter these choke vessel connections, potentially affecting flap viability in secondary procedures [12]. This highlights the importance of thorough preoperative assessment and potential modifications to the surgical technique in patients with previous abdominal scars.

The perforating branches from the deep inferior epigastric system are particularly vital for maintaining the viability of the abdominal flap elevated during abdominoplasty. Extensive undermining can compromise these perforators, increasing the risk of flap ischemia, fat necrosis, and delayed wound healing. Huger's zones of vascularity (Zone I: midline above the umbilicus, Zone II: lateral regions, Zone III: lower abdomen) provide a useful framework for understanding the vascular territories and planning safe dissection in abdominoplasty [13].

Modern imaging techniques, including CT angiography and color Doppler ultrasound, have revolutionized our understanding of abdominal wall perfusion. These technologies allow for preoperative mapping of the dominant perforators, potentially guiding surgical decision-making in complex cases or secondary procedures [14].

Table 2.3: Perforator Distribution Patterns and Surgical Relevance

Location	Typical Number of Dominant Perforators	Average Perforator Diameter	Surgical Significance
Periumbilical region	2–4	1.0–1.5 mm	Critical for central flap viability
Lateral rectus border	3–5 per side	0.7–1.2 mm	Important in high-lateral-tension techniques
Lower abdomen	1–2	0.5–0.8 mm	Often sacrificed during lower incision
Epigastric region	2–3	0.8–1.0 mm	Important in reverse abdominoplasty

Innervation: Sensory Considerations

The sensory innervation of the anterior abdominal wall is a complex interplay of nerves originating from the thoracolumbar region:

1. **Anterior and lateral cutaneous branches of the lower six thoracic nerves (T7–T12)**: These nerves provide the majority of the sensory innervation to the abdominal wall, running between the internal oblique and transversus abdominis muscles before piercing the rectus sheath to supply the overlying skin and subcutaneous tissues.

Table 2.4: Abdominal Wall Sensory Distribution [15, 16]

Nerve	Origin	Area Supplied	Post-abdominoplasty Sensory Changes
T7–T9	Thoracic	Upper abdomen	Minimal sensory deficit
T10–T11	Thoracic	Periumbilical region	Moderate, usually temporary
T12	Thoracic	Lower abdomen	Significant, may persist longer
L1 (iliohypogastric)	Lumbar	Suprapubic region	Often affected, may be permanent
L1 (ilioinguinal)	Lumbar	Groin, upper thigh	Risk with low incisions

2. **First lumbar nerve (L1)**: Contributes to the sensory innervation of the lower abdomen, primarily through its iliohypogastric and ilioinguinal branches.
3. **Iliohypogastric nerve (L1)**: This nerve, after emerging from the lumbar plexus, courses along the iliac crest and provides sensation to the skin of the lower abdomen, upper thigh, and a portion of the external genitalia.
4. **Ilioinguinal nerve (L1)**: This nerve also arises from the lumbar plexus and travels through the inguinal canal alongside the spermatic cord (or round ligament in females), supplying sensation to the skin of the upper medial thigh, scrotum (or labia majora), and the root of the penis (or mons pubis).

Preserving sensory innervation during abdominoplasty is challenging due to the extensive dissection and tissue manipulation involved. However, careful surgical technique, particularly during dissection in the plane between the internal oblique and transversus abdominis muscles, can minimize nerve injury. While some degree of postoperative sensory alteration, including numbness or paresthesia, is often unavoidable in the lower abdomen, these symptoms typically improve over time as nerve regeneration occurs.

Recent studies have demonstrated that 81% of patients report abnormal abdominal skin sensation after abdominoplasty, with the hypogastric region most commonly affected, according to the comprehensive assessment by Presman and colleagues [15]. Studies by Farah and colleagues have shown that sensation gradually returns over 6–18 months, but some degree of sensory alteration may persist, particularly in the lower central abdomen [16]. This information is important for appropriate patient counseling regarding expected outcomes and recovery.

Techniques that limit wide undermining or employ more selective dissection, as seen in some lipoabdominoplasty approaches, may better preserve sensory nerves and result in improved sensory outcomes. Surgeons should consider the balance between adequate flap mobilization and preservation of neurovascular structures when planning their surgical approach.

Clinical implication: Sensory changes

Patients should be specifically counseled about expected sensory changes following abdominoplasty. Explain that numbness in the lower abdomen is nearly universal initially, with gradual improvement over 6–18 months, but some degree of permanent sensory alteration is common. Patients with planned cesarean scars may have preexisting sensory deficits that can be incorporated into your surgical planning, often allowing for the removal of the previously denervated skin.

Lymphatic Drainage: Managing Postoperative Edema and Seroma

The lymphatic system of the abdominal wall plays a vital role in fluid homeostasis and immune function. Disruption of lymphatic drainage during abdominoplasty can contribute to postoperative complications such as prolonged edema, seroma formation, and delayed wound healing. The lymphatic drainage can be broadly divided into superficial and deep networks:

Superficial lymphatics

- **Above the umbilicus:** Lymphatic vessels above the umbilicus generally drain superiorly and laterally toward the axillary lymph nodes.
- **Below the umbilicus:** Lymphatic vessels below the umbilicus drain inferiorly toward the superficial inguinal lymph nodes.

Deep lymphatics

The deep lymphatic vessels generally follow the course of the deep blood vessels, draining to the external iliac, internal iliac, and para-aortic lymph nodes.

Recent lymphosome mapping studies have better delineated the interconnections between superficial and deep lymphatic systems of the abdominal wall [17]. Understanding these connections has informed surgical techniques that better preserve lymphatic integrity.

Surgical techniques that aim to preserve Scarpa's fascia, particularly in the lower abdomen, are thought to help maintain the integrity of the superficial lymphatic network, potentially reducing the incidence of seroma formation and promoting more rapid resolution of postoperative edema. The use of progressive tension sutures (Baroudi sutures), meticulous hemostasis, and appropriate drain management also contribute to minimizing lymphatic complications [18]. Ultrasound studies have demonstrated significantly lower seroma rates in patients where Scarpa's fascia was preserved or where progressive tension sutures were utilized.

Modern approaches to abdominoplasty increasingly emphasize techniques that minimize lymphatic disruption, including selective undermining, preservation of deep fascial attachments when possible, and quilting sutures to obliterate dead space. These modifications have contributed to declining rates of seroma formation in contemporary practice.

Clinical pearl: Lymphatic preservation

To minimize seroma formation, consider:

1. Preserving Scarpa's fascia in the lower abdomen whenever possible
2. Implementing progressive tension sutures to obliterate dead space
3. Maintaining meticulous hemostasis to prevent lymphatic irritation
4. Using closed-suction drains until output is less than 30 mL/24 hr
5. Applying compression garments for at least 4–6 weeks postoperatively.

Diastasis Recti and Its Significance in Abdominoplasty: Restoring Abdominal Wall Integrity

Diastasis recti, a condition characterized by the separation of the rectus abdominis muscles along the linea alba, is a common finding in patients seeking abdominoplasty, particularly in post-partum women or individuals who have experienced significant weight fluctuations. The degree of separation can vary considerably, ranging from a slight widening to a significant gap extending from the xiphoid process to the pubic symphysis.

Classification systems for diastasis recti consider both the width of separation and the length of involvement along the rectus muscles. Supraumbilical diastasis is most common, but infraumbilical or complete diastasis may also be encountered. Asymmetric patterns can present additional challenges for achieving balanced correction.

Correction of diastasis recti through muscle plication is a fundamental component of most abdominoplasty procedures. This involves approximating the medial borders of the rectus muscles by placing a series of sutures along the anterior rectus sheaths, effectively narrowing the waistline, restoring abdominal wall integrity, and improving abdominal contour. The plication can be performed using interrupted or running sutures, and various suture materials can be employed, with non-absorbable or long-lasting absorbable sutures generally preferred for durability. The degree of plication must be carefully calibrated to achieve optimal aesthetic results without causing excessive intra-abdominal pressure or compromising respiratory function. It is important to note that over-tightening can lead to abdominal compartment syndrome in extreme cases.

Studies by Nahas and colleagues provide Level II evidence that rectus muscle plication demonstrates good durability, with most patients maintaining correction at a 10-year follow-up [19]. Tadiparthi and colleagues conducted a systematic review comparing different plication techniques and found that double-layer plication may provide enhanced longevity compared to single-layer techniques, particularly in cases of severe diastasis (Level III evidence) [4]. Some surgeons also advocate for the addition of mesh reinforcement in cases of severe diastasis to enhance the longevity of the repair.

Gender differences in diastasis patterns are increasingly recognized, with men typically presenting with a more focal, supraumbilical separation and with women more commonly exhibiting full-length separation. These differences may influence the approach to plication and overall surgical planning.

Abdominal Wall Hernias: Concurrent Management

While not directly related to the aesthetic goals of abdominoplasty, the identification and management of abdominal wall hernias are important considerations in patients undergoing this procedure. Common types of hernias encountered in this population include:

1. **Umbilical hernias**: These hernias occur through a defect in the abdominal wall at the umbilicus and are often associated with diastasis recti. They may be congenital or acquired and are particularly common in post-pregnancy patients.
2. **Epigastric hernias**: These hernias occur through a defect in the linea alba above the umbilicus and may be asymptomatic or cause pain and discomfort.
3. **Incisional hernias**: These hernias develop at the site of a previous surgical incision where the fascial closure has weakened or broken down over time.
4. **Spigelian hernias**: These are rare hernias occurring along the linea semilunaris, often at the level of the arcuate line or below.

Preoperative identification of hernias is crucial, as they may need to be addressed concurrently with the abdominoplasty procedure. Small hernias can often be repaired primarily, while larger defects may require mesh reinforcement. In some cases, collaboration with a general surgeon may be necessary for optimal management of complex hernias. Failure to address a hernia during abdominoplasty can lead to persistence or worsening of the hernia postoperatively.

Recent advances in combined approaches include the use of laparoscopic hernia repair techniques concurrent with abdominoplasty. A systematic review by Person and colleagues (Level III evidence) has demonstrated that this approach can preserve umbilical vascularization while effectively addressing the hernia [20]. A prospective cohort study (Level II evidence) by Kockerling and colleagues found significantly lower rates of umbilical necrosis with combined laparoscopic approaches compared to traditional open repairs in the setting of abdominoplasty. This is particularly valuable for reducing the risk of umbilical necrosis in patients with umbilical hernias, where traditional open repair might compromise the already tenuous blood supply.

Studies have shown that combined abdominoplasty and hernia repair can be performed safely, though there may be a slightly higher risk of wound complications compared to abdominoplasty alone [21]. Careful patient selection, a meticulous surgical technique, and appropriate postoperative care are essential for successful outcomes in combined procedures.

Clinical pearl: Hernia identification

During preoperative examination, have patients perform a Valsalva maneuver while standing to identify subtle hernias that may be otherwise difficult to detect. During surgery, inspect the entire linea alba and umbilical stalk for small fascial defects that may not have been apparent preoperatively. When repairing umbilical hernias, preserve the periumbilical vasculature by limiting dissection to the hernia sac itself rather than widely mobilizing the entire umbilical stalk.

Modern Technique Advancements

Ongoing refinements in abdominoplasty techniques have incorporated our evolving understanding of abdominal wall anatomy to enhance both aesthetic outcomes and patient safety:

Lipoabdominoplasty

The integration of liposuction with traditional abdominoplasty has revolutionized body contouring approaches. Initially considered high-risk due to concerns about compromising flap vascularity, modern lipoabdominoplasty techniques have proven to be safe and effective when anatomical principles are respected.

Selective undermining approaches preserve perforator vessels, maintaining better flap perfusion than traditional techniques. In a prospective cohort study (Level II evidence), Brauman and colleagues demonstrated that liposuction performed before flap elevation can actually assist with the dissection process while preserving vascular perforators [22]. This finding was corroborated by a systematic review by Swanson (Level III evidence) [23], which showed a reduction in overall complication rates with lipoabdominoplasty compared to traditional techniques. This approach allows for superior contouring results with potentially reduced complication rates.

Key points

- Selective undermining preserves perforator vessels
- Liposuction before flap elevation enhances tissue handling
- Combined approaches allow for more comprehensive contouring
- Preservation of vascular perforators reduces ischemic complications.

High-definition techniques

The pursuit of athletic-appearing results has led to the development of specialized techniques that selectively define underlying muscular anatomy. These approaches require detailed knowledge of the surface projections of underlying muscle groups:

- Selective liposuction along the linea alba and linea semilunaris
- Precise fat preservation over tendinous intersections

- Understanding the anatomical boundaries of the "six-pack" muscular segments
- Recognition of gender-specific differences in ideal muscular definition.

Imaging techniques for surgical planning

Advanced imaging modalities have enhanced our ability to visualize relevant anatomy prior to surgery:

- **CT angiography**: Allows for detailed mapping of perforator vessels, particularly valuable in cases with previous abdominal surgery or complex vascular anatomy [24].
- **Ultrasound evaluation**: Provides real-time assessment of vessel location, diastasis width, and tissue thickness [25].
- **3D imaging**: Facilitates presurgical planning and patient communication regarding expected outcomes.

These technologies supplement clinical examination and can guide surgical decision-making, particularly in challenging cases or revision procedures.

Clinical Implications of Advanced Imaging

While routine imaging is unnecessary for most primary abdominoplasty patients, consider preoperative CT angiography or color Doppler ultrasound in:

1. Patients with multiple previous abdominal surgeries
2. Secondary or revision abdominoplasty cases
3. Patients with compromised vascular status or vasculopathies
4. Cases requiring extensive combined procedures.

These modalities can help identify key perforators to preserve during surgery, potentially reducing flap compromise.

Conclusion: A Foundation for Surgical Excellence

The evolution of abdominoplasty techniques continues to be informed by advances in our understanding of abdominal wall anatomy. From traditional approaches to modern lipoabdominoplasty and high-definition techniques, successful outcomes depend on respecting anatomical principles while embracing innovation. As imaging technology and surgical techniques continue to advance, our ability to preserve critical structures while achieving superior aesthetic results will undoubtedly continue to improve.

This detailed anatomical understanding enables surgeons to perform meticulous dissection, minimize tissue trauma, preserve vital structures, anticipate potential complications, and ultimately achieve superior aesthetic results, restoring both form and function to the abdominal region.

Clinical pearls: Summary

- **Preserve Scarpa's fascia** in the lower abdomen to reduce seroma formation
- **Limit wide-undermining** in the lateral zones to preserve perforator vessels
- **Map vascular perforators** when possible, especially in revision cases
- **Use progressive tension sutures** to reduce dead space and improve lymphatic drainage.

- **Counsel patients** about expected sensory changes, particularly in the hypogastric region.
- **Consider combined laparoscopic approaches** for concurrent hernia repair.

References

1. Costa-Ferreira A, Rebelo M, Vásconez LO, Amarante J. Scarpa fascia preservation during abdominoplasty: A prospective study. *Plast Reconstr Surg.* 2010; **125**(4): 1232–1239. doi:10.1097/PRS.0b013e3181d0a4b0
2. Di Martino M, Nahas FX, Kimura AK, *et al.* Seroma in lipoabdominoplasty and abdominoplasty: A comparative study using ultrasound. *Plast Reconstr Surg.* 2010; **126**(5): 1742–1751. doi:10.1097/PRS.0b013e3181ef8e1c
3. Brauman D, van der Hulst RRWJ, van der Lei B. Liposuction assisted abdominoplasty: An enhanced abdominoplasty technique. *Plast Reconstr Surg Glob Open.* 2018; **6**(9): e1940. doi:10.1097/GOX.0000000000001940
4. Tadiparthi S, Shokrollahi K, Doyle GS, Fahmy FS. Rectus sheath plication in abdominoplasty: Assessment of its longevity and a review of the literature. *J Plast Reconstr Aesthet Surg.* 2012; **65**(3): 328–332. doi:10.1016/j.bjps.2011.09.024
5. van Uchelen JH, Kon M, Werker PM. The long-term durability of plication of the anterior rectus sheath assessed by ultrasonography. *Plast Reconstr Surg.* 2001; **107**(6): 15781584. doi:10.1097/00006534-200105000-00048
6. Centurion P, Olivencia C, Romero C, *et al.* Umbilical reinsertion in abdominoplasty: Technique using deepithelialized skin flaps. *Aesthet Surg J.* 2016; **36**(3): 278–286. doi:10.1093/asj/sjv243
7. Castillo PF, Sepúlveda CA, Prado AC, Troncoso AL, Villamán JJ. Umbilical reinsertion in abdominoplasty: Technique using deepithelialized skin flaps. *Aesthetic Plast Surg.* 2007; **31**(5): 519–520. doi:10.1007/s00266-007-9005-x
8. Rozen WM, Ashton MW, Taylor GI. Reviewing the vascular supply of the anterior abdominal wall: Redefining anatomy for increasingly refined surgery. *Clin Anat.* 2008; **21**(2): 89–98. doi:10.1002/ca.20585
9. El-Mrakby HH, Milner RH. The vascular anatomy of the lower anterior abdominal wall: A microdissection study on the deep inferior epigastric vessels and the perforator branches. *Plast Reconstr Surg.* 2002; **109**(2): 539–543. doi:10.1097/00006534-200202000-00025
10. Rozen WM, Palmer KP, Suami H, *et al.* The DIEA branching pattern and its relationship to perforators: The importance of preoperative computed tomographic angiography for DIEA perforator flaps. *Plast Reconstr Surg.* 2008; **121**(2): 367–373. doi:10.1097/01.prs.0000298315.02712.16
11. Taylor GI, Palmer JH. The vascular territories (angiosomes) of the body: Experimental study and clinical applications. *Br J Plast Surg.* 1987; **40**(2) :113–141. doi:10.1016/0007-1226(87)90185-8
12. Rozen WM, Garcia-Tutor E, Alonso-Burgos A, *et al.* The effect of anterior abdominal wall scars on the vascular anatomy of the abdominal wall: A cadaveric and clinical study with clinical implications. *Clin Anat.* 2009; **22**(7): 815–822. doi:10.1002/ca.20842
13. Huger WE Jr. The anatomic rationale for abdominal lipectomy. *Am Surg.* 1979; **45**(9): 612–617. PMID: 485085
14. Chubb D, Rozen WM, Whitaker IS, Ashton MW. Digital image correlation as a novel method of measuring skin displacement during liposuction of the abdominal wall: Application in the teaching setting. *Aesthetic Plast Surg.* 2011; **35**(6): 963–965. doi:10.1007/s00266-011-9717-9
15. Presman B, Finnerup K, Andresen SR, *et al.* Persistent pain and sensory abnormalities after abdominoplasty. *Plast Reconstr Surg Glob Open.* 2015; **3**(11): e561. doi:10.1097/GOX.0000000000000543
16. Farah AB, Nahas FX, Ferreira LM, *et al.* Sensibility of the abdomen after abdominoplasty. *Plast Reconstr Surg.* 2004; **114**(2): 577–582. doi:10.1097/01.prs.0000128424.86196.89
17. Suami H, Chang DW, Matsumoto K, Kimata Y. Demonstrating the lymphatic system in rats with microinjection. *Anat Rec (Hoboken).* 2011; **294**(9): 1566–1573. doi:10.1002/ar.21450
18. Baroudi R, Ferreira CA. Seroma: How to avoid it and how to treat it. *Aesthet Surg J.* 1998; **18**(6): 439–441. doi:10.1016/S1090-820X(98)70073-1
19. Nahas FX, Ferreira LM, Augusto SM, Ghelfond C. Long-term follow-up of correction of rectus diastasis. *Plast Reconstr Surg.* 2005; **115**(6): 1736–1741. doi:10.1097/01.prs.0000161673.44777.8d
20. Person H, Mojallal A, Braye F, Shipkov H. Techniques of concomitant abdominoplasty and umbilical hernia repair: A review. *Aesthet Surg J.* 2021; **41**(7): NP831-NP839. doi:10.1093/asj/sjaa428
21. Zemlyak AY, Colavita PD, El Djouzi S, *et al.* Comparative study of wound complications: Isolated panniculectomy versus panniculectomy combined with ventral hernia repair. *J Surg Res.* 2012; **177**(2): 387–391. doi:10.1016/j.jss.2012.04.050

22. Brauman D, Capocci J. Liposuction abdominoplasty: An advanced body contouring technique. *Plast Reconstr Surg.* 2018; **141**(2): 369–379. doi:10.1097/PRS.0000000000004121
23. Whitaker IS, Smit JM, Rozen WM, *et al.* Pre- and intraoperative vascular mapping of the lateral thoracic artery perforators for breast reconstruction surgery. *Gland Surg.* 2012; **1**(2): 78–82. doi:10.3978/j.issn.2227-684X.2012.10.03
24. Swanson E. Prospective clinical study reveals significant reduction in triglyceride level and high level of patient satisfaction following lipoabdominoplasty and abdominoplasty. *Plast Reconstr Surg.* 2012; **130**(2): 347e–358e. doi:10.1097/PRS.0b013e318259fdc0
25. Rozen WM, Ribuffo D, Atzeni M, *et al.* Current state of the art in perforator flap imaging with computed tomographic angiography. *Surg Radiol Anat.* 2009; **31**(8): 631–639. doi:10.1007/s00276-009-0525-8

3

Fundamentals of Modern Abdominoplasty

Introduction

Abdominoplasty, commonly known as a "tummy tuck," is a transformative surgical procedure designed to improve the contour and appearance of the abdomen. Patients seeking this procedure present with a diverse range of body types, aesthetic concerns, and functional complaints. Common medical issues include chronic lower back pain, difficulty engaging in physical activities, intertrigo (skin irritation and infections in the abdominal folds), and postural imbalances [1]. Furthermore, a significant proportion of patients express dissatisfaction with their abdominal contour, which can negatively impact self-esteem and body image. This often manifests as the avoidance of swimwear, difficulty finding well-fitting clothing, or a desire to wear more form-fitting attire comfortably.

Historical Evolution of Abdominoplasty: A Journey of Refinement

The field of abdominoplasty has undergone a remarkable evolution, marked by several landmark advancements that have shaped contemporary surgical approaches:

- **Early techniques (late 19th and early 20th centuries)**: Initial abdominoplasty procedures primarily involved simple skin excision, often with limited aesthetic results and significant scarring. Kelly's panniculectomy in 1899 represents one of the earliest documented procedures [2].
- **Pitanguy's contribution (1967)**: Pitanguy's description of a low transverse abdominal incision with wide undermining of the abdominal flap up to the costal margins revolutionized the procedure, allowing for greater skin redraping and improved contour [3].
- **Limited undermining (1977)**: Grazer and Goldwyn advocated for a more conservative approach with limited undermining, demonstrating a reduction in seroma formation [4].
- **High lateral tension abdominoplasty (1995)**: Lockwood's innovative technique, emphasizing high lateral tension with superficial fascial system suspension, significantly improved waistline and flank contouring, addressing a previously challenging area [5].
- **Integration of liposuction (1980s–Present)**: Illouz's pioneering work incorporating liposuction as an adjunct to abdominoplasty further refined abdominal contouring, allowing for more precise fat removal and sculpting [6].
- **Saldanha's lipoabdominoplasty (2001–Present)**: Saldanha and colleagues further refined the integration of liposuction with abdominoplasty, defining the technique of lipoabdominoplasty with selective undermining that preserves more perforator vessels [7].

Table 3.1: Landmark Techniques in Abdominoplasty Evolution

Year	Innovator(s)	Technique	Key Contribution	Limitations
1899	Kelly [2]	Panniculectomy	First documented procedure	Functional focus, limited aesthetic improvement
1967	Pitanguy [3]	Low transverse approach	Standardized technique, improved skin redraping	Extensive undermining, high seroma rates
1977	Grazer and Goldwyn [4]	Limited undermining	Reduced seroma formation	Limited ability to address the upper abdomen
1995	Lockwood [5]	High lateral tension	Enhanced waistline definition	Complex technical demands
2001	Saldanha and colleagues [7]	Lipoabdominoplasty	Preserved vascularity, improved contour	Learning curve, patient selection critical

Modern Abdominoplasty Techniques: A Spectrum of Approaches

Today, a diverse array of abdominoplasty techniques exists, encompassing both novel approaches and modifications of established methods. These techniques often combine varying degrees of:

- **Muscle plication**: Tightening and repair of the abdominal muscles, particularly the rectus abdominis.
- **Skin excision**: Removal of excess skin.
- **Liposuction**: Targeted fat removal for enhanced contouring.

Despite the wide range of techniques available, patients with significant skin laxity, marked diastasis recti (separation of the rectus abdominis muscles exceeding 2–3 cm), and substantial lipodystrophy (abnormal fat distribution) can present unique challenges requiring customized approaches.

Clinical pearl: Technique selection

When selecting an abdominoplasty technique, consider these key factors:

1. **Skin quality and elasticity**—poor elasticity requires more aggressive resection
2. **Degree and pattern of diastasis recti**—complete separation may require extended plication
3. **Fat distribution**—localized deposits benefit from combined liposuction
4. **Previous scars**—may dictate flap design and undermining extent
5. **Patient goals and lifestyle**—athletic patients may benefit from high-definition techniques.

Principles of Modern Abdominoplasty: A Multifaceted Approach

Modern abdominoplasty is characterized by meticulous preoperative planning, precise surgical execution, and a comprehensive approach that often integrates multiple modalities to achieve optimal outcomes. It typically involves:

- **Rectus muscle plication**: Correction of diastasis recti and restoration of abdominal wall integrity. Long-term studies have demonstrated the durability of this repair, with maintained correction at a 10+-year follow-up [8].
- **Excision of excess skin and fat**: Tailored removal of redundant tissue to create a smoother, flatter abdominal contour.

- **Liposuction:** Strategic fat removal to enhance contouring, particularly in the flanks and upper abdomen. This may be performed before, during, or after the excisional portion of the procedure, depending on the specific technique employed.
- **Scar placement:** Low transverse incision designed to be concealed by most underwear or swimwear, although the final scar appearance can vary depending on individual healing factors.

Detailed Anatomical Considerations and Surgical Steps

Upper abdomen

The upper abdominal skin flap is typically elevated superiorly to the level of the xiphoid process (the lower tip of the sternum) and laterally to the costal margins. This extensive undermining provides access to the entire length of the rectus abdominis muscles, enabling comprehensive plication from the xiphoid to the pubis. It also facilitates redistribution and redraping of the abdominal skin.

Care must be taken during dissection to preserve the delicate perforating blood vessels, especially those emanating from the deep inferior epigastric system, which are crucial for maintaining flap viability [9]. In more recent modifications, such as lipoabdominoplasty, selective undermining is employed to preserve more perforators, potentially reducing the risk of flap ischemia and related complications.

Lower abdomen

The lower abdomen is the primary site of skin and fat excision. The lower incision is strategically placed low on the abdomen, typically within the natural skin crease just superior to the pubic region and extending laterally toward the anterior superior iliac spines. This low placement is designed to conceal the eventual scar beneath most types of underwear or swimwear.

The amount of tissue excised is determined intraoperatively after muscle plication and lateral tension sutures, allowing for precise tailoring of the abdominal contour. This approach minimizes the risk of excessive or inadequate tissue removal, which could result in either residual laxity or excessive tension at the closure.

Clinical pearl: Lower incision placement

The optimal lower incision placement should:

1. Follow natural skin creases (typically 7–8 cm above the vulvar commissure in women)
2. Remain within the bikini/underwear line (assess the patient's preferred style)
3. Curve gently upward laterally toward the ASIS
4. Be placed higher in patients with significant lower abdominal laxity to avoid pubic distortion
5. Take into account pre-existing scars when possible.

Multi-Level Abdominal Wall Support: A Layered Reconstruction

The concept of multi-level abdominal wall support emphasizes a layered approach to reconstruction, mimicking the natural anatomy and providing structural integrity:

Base level (muscular layer)

- Plication of the rectus abdominis muscles, typically using a strong, non-absorbable (e.g., polypropylene) or long-lasting absorbable (e.g., polydioxanone) running suture

- Extends from the xiphoid process to the pubic symphysis
- Corrects diastasis recti, narrows the waistline
- Newer modifications include a double-breasted plication technique for enhanced reinforcement
- Research has shown properly performed muscle plication maintains its correction, with studies demonstrating stability at a 10+-year follow-up [8]

Intermediate level (Scarpa's fascia)

- Careful management of Scarpa's fascia, a distinct membranous layer within subcutaneous tissue
- Some techniques involve suturing Scarpa's fascia to deeper muscular fascia or anterior rectus sheath
- Studies have demonstrated a significantly lower rate of seroma formation when Scarpa's fascia is preserved in the lower abdomen [10]
- This preservation may maintain lymphatic drainage channels, facilitating more efficient fluid absorption postoperatively

Superficial level (skin redraping)

- Meticulous redraping of the abdominal skin flap, ensuring smooth contours and appropriate tension
- Progressive tension sutures (Pollock sutures) distribute tension more evenly across the abdominal flap
- Minimizes tension at the incision line, potentially improving scar quality
- Reduces dead space and seroma formation [11].

Umbilical Transposition: Restoring the Aesthetic Centerpiece

The umbilicus is a critical aesthetic landmark of the abdomen. Its position and appearance significantly contribute to the overall abdominal contour. During abdominoplasty, the umbilicus is typically detached from the abdominal skin flap and later transposed to a new, aesthetically pleasing position.

This new position is generally at or slightly inferior to the level of the iliac crests, approximately at 61–67% of the xiphoid-pubic distance [12]. This specific measurement represents the most natural-appearing position based on anthropometric studies of aesthetically pleasing umbilical placement. The measurement is taken from the xiphoid process to the pubic symphysis, with the umbilicus ideally positioned at approximately two-thirds of this distance from the xiphoid.

The final position is best determined after the abdominal wall reconstruction is complete and the patient is placed in a semi-sitting position. This allows for an accurate assessment of the natural drape of the skin and the most harmonious umbilical location. Various techniques exist for umbilical transposition, including those that create a circular, oval, or inverted-V-shaped incision around the umbilicus. Different suturing techniques are employed to create a natural-looking umbilical depression and minimize scarring.

Modern techniques focus on creating an appropriately sized, vertically oriented umbilicus with a slight superior hood to achieve the most natural-appearing result. Attention to these details can significantly enhance the overall aesthetic outcome of the procedure.

Clinical pearl: Umbilical transposition

For optimal umbilical aesthetics:

1. Position the new umbilicus at 61–67% of the xiphoid-pubic distance
2. Create a vertical, slightly oval (rather than perfectly round) orientation

3. Ensure a natural superior hood by preserving dermal attachments superiorly
4. Avoid excessive tension around the stalk to maintain adequate blood supply
5. Consider deepithelialized flaps for creating natural contour and minimizing visible scars.

Tension-Free Skin Closure: Promoting Optimal Scarring

Skin elasticity varies considerably among individuals and is influenced by factors such as age, genetics, sun exposure, and history of pregnancy or weight fluctuations. Techniques that rely heavily on skin tension to maintain abdominal contour often yield less durable results, with a higher likelihood of early recurrence of skin laxity. Conversely, excessive tension can compromise wound healing, leading to wound dehiscence, widened scars, and hypertrophic or keloid scar formation.

Modern abdominoplasty emphasizes minimizing tension on the final skin closure. This is achieved through:

- **Careful preoperative planning and markings**: Accurate assessment of skin laxity and precise markings guide the extent of skin excision.
- **Comprehensive muscle plication**: Adequate tightening of the abdominal muscles reduces the reliance on skin tension for contouring.
- **Progressive tension sutures**: These sutures, placed strategically within the deeper layers of the abdominal flap, help to distribute tension evenly across the wound, reducing tension at the skin edges [11].

Alternative scar management strategies may include:

- Silicone-based scar products (sheets, gels) beginning 2–3 weeks postoperatively
- Fractional laser treatments for mature scars with persistent erythema or hypertrophy
- Intralesional steroid injections for early hypertrophic scar formation
- Compression garments during the early healing phase.

Table 3.2: Scar Management Strategies by Timeline

Timing	Intervention	Mechanism	Evidence Level
0–3 weeks	Taping, silicone-based dressings	Prevent tension, hydration	II
3 weeks to 3 months	Silicone sheets/gels, compression	Hydration, pressure, reduced tension	I
3–6 months	Corticosteroid injections*	Anti-inflammatory, collagen reduction	II
>6 months	Fractional laser therapy	Collagen remodeling	II

*For hypertrophic or keloid tendency only.

Goals of Abdominoplasty: A Holistic Perspective

The overarching goals of abdominoplasty encompass both aesthetic and functional improvements:

Primary goals

- **Safe and reproducible results**: Consistent outcomes with a low complication rate
- **Correction of muscle laxity**: Repair of diastasis recti and restoration of abdominal wall integrity
- **Removal of excess skin**: Elimination of redundant skin and improvement of abdominal contour
- **Improvement of abdominal contour**: Creation of a smoother, flatter, and more aesthetically pleasing abdominal profile

- **Limited and favorable scarring**: Strategically placed and meticulously closed incisions to minimize scar visibility
- **Preservation of sensation**: Minimizing nerve disruption during dissection to preserve abdominal wall sensation where possible
- **Improvement in functional symptoms**: Alleviation of back pain, improvement in posture, and enhanced core strength.

Secondary goals

- **Easily learnable technique**: A procedure that can be readily mastered by surgeons with the appropriate training.
- **Amenability to secondary operations**: The ability to perform revisions or additional procedures if needed.
- **Adaptable markings and technique**: Flexibility to customize the procedure to different body types and varying degrees of deformity.

Symmetry, Scars, Safety, Stability, and Sensitivity: The Five Pillars of Success

Symmetry

Achieving symmetry is a fundamental goal in abdominoplasty. The amount of skin excised is typically determined intraoperatively after muscle plication and abdominal wall reconstruction are complete. This allows for a more accurate assessment of symmetry and enables adjustments to be made as needed to ensure a balanced and harmonious result. The final position of the umbilicus is also crucial for symmetry and is carefully evaluated before the final closure.

Scars

Minimizing the visibility of scars is a paramount concern for patients undergoing abdominoplasty. The low transverse incision is strategically placed to be concealed by most types of underwear or swimwear. However, individual healing factors can influence the final scar appearance. Techniques that minimize tension on the incision, such as comprehensive muscle plication and the use of progressive tension sutures, are essential for promoting the formation of thin, inconspicuous scars.

Safety

Patient safety is of utmost importance in any surgical procedure. Meticulous surgical technique, careful patient selection, and appropriate management of medical comorbidities are crucial for minimizing complications. Strategies to reduce the risk of deep vein thrombosis (DVT) and pulmonary embolism (PE) are employed, including the use of sequential compression devices (SCDs), early ambulation, and in selected high-risk cases, chemoprophylaxis [13].

Appropriate patient selection is crucial, with particular attention to the body mass index (BMI), comorbidities, and smoking status, as these factors significantly impact complication rates. Studies have highlighted the increased risk of complications in obese patients undergoing abdominoplasty, emphasizing the importance of careful patient selection and risk stratification [13].

Stability

Multi-level abdominal wall reconstruction, encompassing muscle plication, Scarpa's fascia management, and meticulous skin redraping, is designed to provide long-lasting results. This layered approach not only creates an aesthetically pleasing contour but also recreates the necessary fascial support to maintain a stable abdominal shape over time.

Furthermore, patients are counseled on the importance of maintaining a healthy lifestyle, including a balanced diet and regular exercise, to optimize and preserve their surgical results. Long-term studies have demonstrated the durability of properly performed muscle plication, with maintained correction at a 10+-year follow-up [8].

Sensitivity

While complete preservation of abdominal wall sensation is not always possible due to the necessary division of sensory nerves during flap elevation, efforts are made to minimize nerve disruption. Careful dissection in the appropriate planes and identification of major sensory nerves can help to preserve sensation where possible.

Postoperatively, patients may experience areas of numbness or altered sensation, particularly in the lower abdomen, but these typically improve over time as nerve regeneration occurs. Studies have shown progressive improvement in sensation over 6–18 months postoperatively, although some degree of sensory alteration may persist indefinitely [14].

Clinical pearl: Patient counseling on sensory changes

Inform patients that:

1. Altered sensation or numbness in the lower abdomen is normal and expected
2. Improvement typically begins at the periphery and progresses centrally
3. Most sensation recovers within 6–18 months
4. Some degree of permanent sensory change in the lower central abdomen is common
5. These changes rarely affect normal activities or quality of life.

Complication Rates in Abdominoplasty

Table 3.3: Comparison of Complication Rates from Key Studies

Complication	Standard Abdominoplasty (%)	Lipoabdominoplasty (%)	Massive Weight Loss Patients (%)	References
Seroma	10–15	5–8	15–25	[10, 15]
Hematoma	2–5	1–3	3–8	[4, 13]
Infection	3–5	2–4	5–10	[13, 15]
Wound dehiscence	5–10	3–7	10–20	[13]
DVT/PE	0.5–1	0.3–0.8	1–3	[13, 15]
Skin necrosis	2–5	1–3	5–10	[4, 13]
Persistent sensory changes	70–80	60–75	80–90	[14]
Scar hypertrophy	10–15	8–12	15–25	[15]

Note: Ranges represent approximate values from multiple studies. Individual surgeon experience and patient factors may influence actual rates.

Functional Improvement: Beyond Aesthetics

Abdominoplasty, particularly when combined with rectus muscle plication, can lead to significant functional improvements. Studies have demonstrated improvements in:

- **Back pain**: Strengthening the abdominal muscles can improve core stability and reduce strain on the lower back, leading to a reduction in chronic back pain. In a prospective study of 214 patients, Carter and Janssen [1] reported a 78% reduction in pre-existing back pain symptoms at a 6-month follow-up.
- **Urinary incontinence**: In some cases, abdominoplasty with muscle plication may improve stress urinary incontinence by providing support to the pelvic floor. According to Carter and Janssen [1], 62% of patients with pre-existing stress urinary incontinence reported significant improvement following abdominoplasty with rectus plication.
- **Core strength**: Tightening the abdominal muscles enhances core strength and stability, improving posture, balance, and overall physical function. Objective measurements showed an average of 35% improvement in core muscle strength at 3 months postoperatively [1].

Recent research has increasingly focused on these functional benefits, highlighting abdominoplasty as not merely an aesthetic procedure but one with significant quality-of-life improvements for patients [1].

Adaptability: Tailoring the Procedure to Individual Needs

Modern abdominoplasty techniques are highly adaptable and can be customized to address a wide spectrum of abdominal contour concerns, ranging from mild skin laxity to the significant deformities seen in massive weight loss patients. The use of individualized markings, tailored skin excision after abdominal wall reconstruction, and the integration of liposuction allow the surgeon to adapt the procedure to each patient's unique anatomy and aesthetic goals.

For massive weight loss patients, specialized classification systems such as the Pittsburgh Rating Scale can help to standardize the assessment of deformities and guide the selection of appropriate surgical techniques [16]. These patients often require more extensive procedures, potentially incorporating flank and lateral thigh contouring as well.

This versatility makes abdominoplasty a powerful tool for addressing a broad range of body contouring challenges, from the post-pregnancy patient seeking restoration of pre-pregnancy contours to the massive weight loss patient requiring comprehensive reconstruction.

Clinical pearl: Surgical planning

For optimal surgical planning:

1. Take standardized photographs from multiple angles (front, lateral, oblique)
2. Mark patients in a standing position to accurately assess tissue laxity
3. Discuss aesthetic and functional goals to establish priorities
4. Consider complementary procedures (e.g., liposuction, hernia repair)
5. Develop contingency plans for intraoperative findings that may alter the approach.

Conclusion: A Comprehensive and Evolving Approach

Abdominoplasty has evolved from a simple skin excision procedure to a sophisticated and multifaceted operation that addresses both aesthetic and functional concerns. Modern techniques emphasize a comprehensive approach, incorporating muscle plication, tailored skin and fat removal, and meticulous attention to detail.

By adhering to the principles of multi-level abdominal wall reconstruction, minimizing tension on the skin closure, and prioritizing patient safety, surgeons can achieve consistently excellent outcomes, restoring both form and function to the abdomen while minimizing complications and optimizing patient satisfaction.

The ongoing refinement of techniques and the integration of adjunctive procedures like liposuction continue to enhance the transformative potential of abdominoplasty, solidifying its role as a cornerstone of body contouring surgery. Future directions may include further refinements in selective undermining techniques, enhanced understanding of the functional benefits of abdominoplasty, and improved scar management strategies, all contributing to even better outcomes for patients.

References

1. Papadopulos NA, Staffler V, Mirceva V, *et al.* Does abdominoplasty have a positive influence on quality of life, self-esteem, and emotional stability? *Plast Reconstr Surg.* 2012; **129**(6): 957e–962e. doi:10.1097/PRS.0b013e31824e2a0a
2. Kelly HA. Report of gynaecological cases. *Johns Hopkins Hospital Bulletin.* 1899; **10**: 197.
3. Pitanguy I. Abdominal lipectomy: An approach to it through an analysis of 300 consecutive cases. *Plast Reconstr Surg.* 1967; **40**(4): 384–391. doi:10.1097/00006534-196710000-00001
4. Grazer FM, Goldwyn RM. Abdominoplasty assessed by survey. *Plast Reconstr Surg.* 1977; **59**(4): 513–517. doi:10.1097/00006534-197704000-00001
5. Lockwood T. High-lateral-tension abdominoplasty with superficial fascial system suspension. *Plast Reconstr Surg.* 1995; **96**(3): 603–615. doi:10.1097/00006534-199509000-00010
6. Illouz YG. Body contouring by lipolysis: A 5-year experience with over 3000 cases. *Plast Reconstr Surg.* 1983; **72**(5): 591–597. doi:10.1097/00006534-198311000-00001
7. Saldanha OR, De Souza Pinto EB, Mattos WN Jr, *et al.* Lipoabdominoplasty with selective and safe undermining. *Aesthetic Plast Surg.* 2003; **27**(4): 322–327. doi:10.1007/s00266-003-3027-5
8. Nahas FX, Ferreira LM, Augusto SM, Ghelfond C. Long-term follow-up of correction of rectus diastasis. *Plast Reconstr Surg.* 2005; **115**(6): 1736–1741. doi:10.1097/01.prs.0000161673.44777.8d
9. El-Mrakby HH, Milner RH. The vascular anatomy of the lower anterior abdominal wall: A microdissection study. *Plast Reconstr Surg.* 2002; **109**(2): 539–543. doi:10.1097/00006534-200202000-00025
10. Costa-Ferreira A, Rebelo M, Vásconez LO, Amarante J. Scarpa fascia preservation during abdominoplasty: A prospective study. *Plast Reconstr Surg.* 2010; **125**(4): 1232–1239. doi:10.1097/PRS.0b013e3181d0a4b0
11. Pollock H, Pollock T. Progressive tension sutures: A technique to reduce local complications in abdominoplasty. *Plast Reconstr Surg.* 2000; **105**(7): 2583–2586. doi:10.1097/00006534-200006000-00023
12. Castillo PF, Sepúlveda CA, Prado AC, *et al.* Umbilical reinsertion in abdominoplasty: Technique using deepithelialized skin flaps. *Aesthetic Plast Surg.* 2007; **31**(5): 519–520. doi:10.1007/s00266-007-9005-x
13. Momeni A, Heier M, Bannasch H, Stark GB. Complications in abdominoplasty: A risk factor analysis. *J Plast Reconstr Aesthet Surg.* 2009; **62**(10): 1250–1254. doi:10.1016/j.bjps.2008.07.019

4

Patient Consultation and Evaluation for Abdominoplasty

Introduction

The success of an abdominoplasty procedure hinges not only on surgical skill but also on a comprehensive preoperative consultation and evaluation process. While a plastic surgeon may dedicate more time to marketing efforts than to surgery itself in private practice, the consultation should never be treated like a sales pitch. Unlike a car salesman who highlights only the positive attributes of their product, a plastic surgeon has an ethical obligation to thoroughly educate patients about the potential benefits, limitations, risks, and alternatives to the procedure. This includes candidly discussing potential drawbacks, such as the possibility of scar formation, sensory changes, and the potential for some degree of recurrence of skin laxity over time, even with optimal surgical technique.

The consultation process is particularly important when discussing the multi-level abdominoplasty technique, as patients need to understand how this approach differs from traditional methods and why its comprehensive, layered reconstruction offers superior structural integrity and potentially longer-lasting results.

Key Points

- Thorough consultation is essential for patient selection, expectation management, and surgical planning.
- Understanding patient motivations helps predict satisfaction with outcomes.
- Proper identification of psychological red flags reduces postoperative dissatisfaction.
- Systematic physical examination guides technique selection and individualization.
- Comprehensive documentation supports informed consent and medicolegal protection.

Understanding Patient Motivations and Setting Realistic Expectations

Prior to formulating a treatment plan, it is imperative to delve into the patient's motivations for seeking abdominal contouring and to thoroughly assess their expectations. A frank and open discussion is necessary to ensure that the patient's goals are realistic and surgically attainable. It is essential to ascertain the patient's desired abdominal appearance. Unrealistic expectations, such as achieving a perfectly flat abdomen or a "six-pack" in every case, must be addressed and modified.

The surgical plan should aim to provide the patient with an optimal abdominal shape while minimizing scarring and considering the patient's individual anatomy and goals. Rohrich and colleagues [1] emphasized the importance of managing patient expectations in body contouring procedures, highlighting that a clear understanding of achievable outcomes is crucial for patient satisfaction.

With the multi-level abdominoplasty technique, it is important to explain to patients that while the procedure may be more comprehensive than some alternatives, it offers the advantage of addressing multiple anatomical components (muscle, fascia, and skin) in a single operation, potentially yielding more harmonious and durable results.

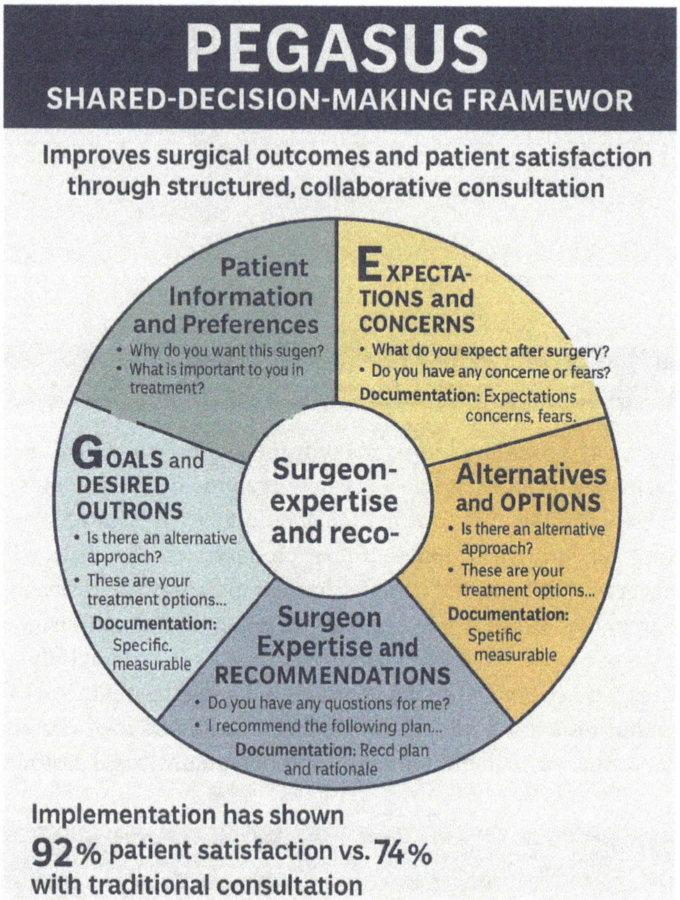

Figure 4.1. ■ **PEGASUS shared-decision-making wheel.** Schematic of the PEGASUS conversation model used in abdominoplasty consultations. The seven spokes—Patient Information and Preferences, Expectations and Concerns, Alternatives and Options, Surgeon Expertise and Recommendations, and Goals and Desired Outcomes—anchor the discussion around the surgeon's judgment at the hub. When applied as written in this chapter, the tool pushed satisfaction to 92 % versus 74 % for unstructured visits, proving that structured dialogue beats ad-hoc salesmanship every time.

The Consultation Process: A Deep Dive into Patient Needs

Motivations and indications: Why now?

The initial phase of the consultation involves exploring the patient's reasons for seeking abdominoplasty at this particular juncture in their life. Understanding the "why now" is crucial for gauging the patient's emotional readiness and the stability of their decision-making process.

Younger patients

For younger patients, the motivation is often straightforward: they may seek treatment as soon as they can afford it or after completing their families. They are typically concerned about excess skin and fat, often resulting from pregnancy or weight fluctuations. However, they may not fully appreciate the potential for postoperative pain, the nature of scarring, or the possibility of changes in abdominal sensation.

Younger patients with minimal skin laxity often harbor high expectations for a flawless result. However, their generally firmer skin may be predisposed to more noticeable scarring, including hypertrophic scars or keloids. Therefore, meticulous surgical technique, careful scar placement, and comprehensive postoperative scar management are paramount in this group. Vercler and colleagues [2] described genetic testing for keloid predisposition, which can be particularly valuable for younger patients with family histories of abnormal scarring. While these genetic markers (including polymorphisms in the NEDD4 and FOXL2 genes) show promise in identifying high-risk patients, it should be noted that clinical implementation remains limited, with current utility primarily in research settings rather than routine preoperative screening.

The multi-level abdominoplasty technique is particularly beneficial for younger post-pregnancy patients who often present with both skin laxity and significant diastasis recti. The technique's emphasis on thorough muscle plication from the xiphoid to the pubis creates a strong internal foundation that supports the abdominal contour, reducing the reliance on skin tension for maintaining shape.

Older Patients or Those with Significant Skin Laxity

Diverse factors motivate older patients or those with significant skin laxity. Matarasso and colleagues [3] found that this group often delays seeking treatment due to childcare responsibilities, financial constraints, or the need to achieve stable weight loss. Interestingly, their motivation is often less purely aesthetic and more driven by functional concerns. These can include difficulty finding well-fitting clothes, skin irritation or infections (intertrigo) in redundant abdominal folds, and limitations in physical activity.

While concerned about postoperative shape and scar appearance, they often express a desire for improved core strength and may have more realistic expectations regarding the degree of aesthetic improvement, as supported by van der Beek and colleagues [4].

The multi-level abdominoplasty approach is especially valuable for this patient group, as it addresses both aesthetic and functional concerns. The comprehensive muscle plication can significantly improve core strength and posture, while the layered closure system provides the structural support needed to maintain results in patients with compromised tissue elasticity.

Massive Weight Loss Patients

Individuals who have undergone massive weight loss, either through lifestyle modifications or bariatric surgery, represent a unique patient population. They often present with extensive skin laxity and redundancy, not only in the abdomen but also in other body areas. While they typically have realistic expectations due to their transformative weight loss journey, they require careful counseling regarding the potential need for multiple staged procedures to address excess skin comprehensively.

They should be informed about the limitations of surgery in achieving their ideal body contour and the importance of long-term weight maintenance, as outlined by Rubin and colleagues [5].

For massive weight loss patients, the multi-level abdominoplasty technique offers distinct advantages, particularly its ability to provide robust internal support through comprehensive muscle plication and fascial reinforcement. This is crucial for patients whose tissues have been significantly compromised by extreme weight fluctuations. The multi-level approach helps distribute tension evenly across the abdominal wall, potentially reducing the risk of recurrent laxity in this challenging patient population.

Key Characteristics of Three Main Abdominoplasty Patient Groups

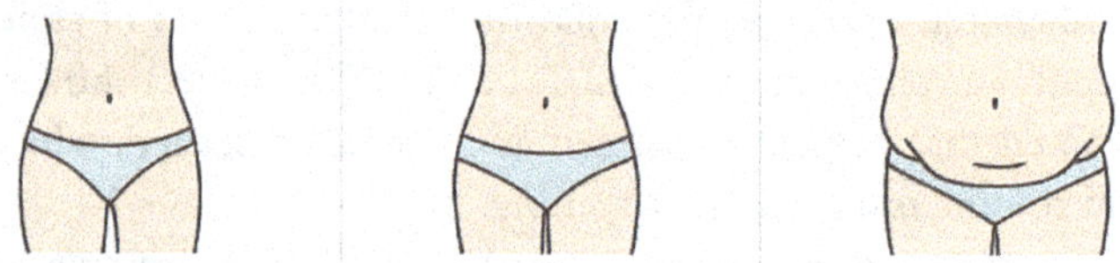

Younger Post-Pregnancy Patients	Older Patients with Skin Laxity	Massive Weight Loss Patients
Primary Motivation Postpartum contour improvement	Skin tightening Contour enhancment	Removal of redundant tissue, contour resorat-ion
Typical Anatomical Presentation	Mild to moderate skin laxity Minimal striae	Severe skin laxity Significant pannus
Expectation (realistic vs. unrealistic)	Striae improvement Improved laxity vs minimal scars. Skin appearance akin to youth	Scar camoutlage Complete restoration
Key Concerns Stretch marks Diastasis recti	Scar placement Residual laxity	Wound healing Malnutrition
Psychological Considerationns	Acceptance of aging process	Improvement in body image

Figure 4.2. ■ Three prototypical abdominoplasty phenotypes. Side-by-side infographic contrasting the clinical and psychological hallmarks of (A) younger post-pregnancy patients, (B) older patients with progressive skin laxity, and (C) massive weight loss patients. Primary motivations, anatomical patterns, expectations, key concerns, and mindset red-flags are distilled into a single glance. Use this grid to match technique—including the multi-level approach—to the patient in front of you rather than forcing every abdomen into the same mold.

Psychological Considerations: Identifying Red Flags

A thorough discussion about the patient's motivations and expectations can reveal important psychological factors that may influence their suitability for surgery and their postoperative satisfaction. Utilizing structured assessment tools such as the PEGASUS framework (Patient Expectations, Goals, and Added value in Shared Understanding for Surgery) can facilitate this process, as demonstrated by Ridgway and colleagues [6], who found improved patient satisfaction rates of 92% versus 74% in traditional consultations when using structured shared decision-making tools.

Clinical pearl: Structured patient assessment

The PEGASUS framework for comprehensive patient evaluation includes:

1. **P**atient history (medical, surgical, psychological)
2. **E**xpectations assessment (specific goals and timeline)
3. **G**oals clarification (realistic vs. unrealistic)
4. **A**lternatives discussion (non-surgical options)
5. **S**upport system evaluation (recovery assistance)
6. **U**nderstanding verification (knowledge of limitations)
7. **S**tability assessment (life circumstances, emotional state)

Implementing this structured approach has been shown to improve satisfaction rates by 18% in prospective studies [6].

Stable vs. Unstable Motivations

Patients who have experienced significant weight loss or completed childbearing and have no plans for future pregnancies often have well-considered motivations. They typically have strong family support, realistic expectations, and an understanding that scars will take time to mature and that the results may evolve with aging or weight fluctuations, as noted by Rohrich and colleagues [1].

Patients Undergoing Life Stressors

In contrast, patients experiencing abrupt and stressful life changes, such as divorce, job loss, or the death of a loved one, may seek immediate and dramatic improvements through surgery. While some may have carefully considered their decision, others may act impulsively. These individuals may not be psychologically prepared for the postoperative recovery period or the gradual evolution of the surgical results.

They may be overly critical of minor imperfections in scars or shape and may be more prone to dissatisfaction, especially if complications arise. Sarwer and colleagues [7] highlighted the importance of assessing psychological factors in cosmetic surgery patients, as those undergoing significant life stress may have less stable motivations. Surgeons should be attuned to these patients' emotional states and proceed cautiously. It is often prudent to postpone surgery until the patient's life circumstances are more stable.

Unrealistic Expectations

Patients with unrealistic expectations require careful evaluation and counseling. Some may have been previously advised by another surgeon that liposuction alone could address their concerns. While liposuction is less invasive, it is often insufficient for patients with significant skin laxity or muscle diastasis.

It can be challenging to explain the need for a more extensive procedure that inevitably involves scarring. These patients may mistakenly believe that their abdominal protrusion is solely due to fat and may not comprehend the need to address skin and muscle laxity surgically. As Matarasso and Wallach [8] discussed, patient education is key to managing expectations regarding the limitations of liposuction alone in cases of significant skin laxity.

When discussing the multi-level abdominoplasty technique with these patients, it is important to emphasize that while it may involve more extensive dissection compared to some alternatives, this approach enables the surgeon to address all components of abdominal deformity—muscle laxity, fascial weakness, and skin redundancy—in a single procedure. This comprehensive approach often yields superior three-dimensional contouring that cannot be achieved with liposuction alone.

Minimally Invasive Options

Conversely, some patients with minimal skin laxity may request a full abdominoplasty when less invasive options like a mini-abdominoplasty or liposuction alone might be more appropriate. It is important to educate these patients that a full abdominoplasty in such cases might be unnecessarily aggressive, resulting in a more extensive scar than warranted by the degree of improvement.

The multi-level abdominoplasty technique can be adapted to varying degrees of deformity, and for patients with minimal laxity, a modified approach with more limited dissection may be appropriate. This adaptability allows the surgeon to tailor the procedure to each patient's unique needs while still applying the principles of comprehensive structural support.

External Pressures

Individuals who seek surgery primarily to please a partner rather than for their own intrinsic desire should be discouraged. Their motivations are often not well-founded, and they may later regret their decision.

Body Dysmorphic Disorder

Patients who express excessive concern about minor or perceived flaws in their appearance may have body dysmorphic disorder (BDD). These individuals often have unrealistic expectations and may never be satisfied with the results of surgery. They may focus on perceived imperfections that are not objectively noticeable. Surgeons should be vigilant for signs of BDD and consider referral to a mental health professional when appropriate, as highlighted by Sarwer and colleagues [7].

Table 4.1: Red Flags During Patient Assessment

Category	Warning Signs	Recommended Action
Psychological	History of untreated depression/anxiety	Consider mental health referral
	Multiple cosmetic procedures with dissatisfaction	Psychological evaluation before proceeding
	Excessive focus on minor imperfections	Screen for body dysmorphic disorder
Motivational	Recent major life event (divorce, death, etc.)	Consider postponing surgery
	External pressure from others	Ensure the patient's autonomous decision
	Expectation of life transformation	Clarify realistic outcome scope
Expectations	Desire for "perfect" result	Set realistic limits on the outcome
	Insistence on minimal scarring	Detailed illustration of scar location/development
	Unwillingness to accept potential complications	Defer surgery until properly informed

Contraindications: Recognizing When to Say No

While most patients are suitable candidates for abdominoplasty, certain contraindications should be considered:

Psychological contraindications

- **Unrealistic expectations**: As previously discussed, patients with unrealistic expectations may not be suitable candidates.
- **Body dysmorphic disorder**: Patients with BDD should be carefully evaluated and may require psychological intervention before considering surgery.
- **Unstable psychological state**: Patients experiencing significant life stressors or emotional instability may not be ideal candidates.
- **Desire for perfection**: Patients seeking an unattainable "perfect" result should be counseled about the limitations of surgery.
- **Minor deformities**: Patients with very minor abdominal contour irregularities may not derive sufficient benefit from abdominoplasty to justify the scars and recovery.

Medical contraindications

- **Active skin infections or intertrigo**: These conditions should be treated and resolved before surgery.
- **Uncontrolled medical conditions**: While conditions like hypertension, diabetes, and lung diseases are not absolute contraindications, they should be well-controlled preoperatively to minimize surgical risk. Careful evaluation and optimization by the patient's primary care physician or specialist are essential. As Hensel and colleagues [9] reported, patients with well-managed comorbidities can undergo abdominoplasty safely.
- **High body mass index (BMI)**: Patients with an elevated BMI have an increased risk of complications. The following table summarizes the recommended approach based on BMI categories:

Table 4.2: BMI Considerations and Risk Stratification

BMI Category	Complication Risk	Recommended Action	Specific Complication Rate
<30	Low	Proceed	8–12% overall [10]
30–35	Moderate	Weight loss encouraged	18–24% overall [10, 11]
>35	High	Delay until BMI ≤30	32–45% overall [10, 12]

Hasanbegovic and Sorensen [10] found significantly higher complication rates in patients with BMI >35 undergoing abdominoplasty (45% vs. 12% in BMI <30 patients), with specific increases in seroma formation (32% vs. 7%) and wound dehiscence (22% vs. 4%). These findings confirm earlier results by Vastine and colleagues [12] and provide quantitative risk assessment for patient counseling.

Clinical pearl: Comorbidity management

For optimal patient preparation:

1. Diabetes should be controlled with HbA1c <7.0%
2. Blood pressure consistently <140/90 mmHg
3. Smoking cessation at least 4 weeks before and after surgery
4. BMI optimization to <30 when possible, with careful risk stratification for BMI 30–35
5. Nutritional assessment in massive weight loss patients (albumin >3.5 g/dL, pre-albumin >20 mg/dL).

Document all recommendations and patient compliance in the medical record.

Medical History and Physical Examination: A Comprehensive Assessment

A thorough medical history and physical examination are essential components of the preoperative evaluation:

Medical history

- **Personal and family history**: Inquire about any medical conditions, previous surgeries, allergies, medications, and family history of medical problems, particularly bleeding disorders or adverse reactions to anesthesia.
- **Pregnancy and childbearing history**: Document the number of pregnancies, type of deliveries (vaginal or cesarean), and any complications. Inquire about future pregnancy plans, as this can impact the surgical plan and long-term results.
- **Weight history**: Obtain a detailed weight history, including maximum and minimum adult weights, recent weight fluctuations, and any history of massive weight loss.
- **Lifestyle factors**: Assess smoking status, alcohol consumption, and exercise habits. Smoking significantly increases the risk of complications and should be strongly discouraged for at least 4 weeks before and after surgery.
- **Psychological history**: Inquire about any history of mental health conditions, such as depression, anxiety, or eating disorders.

Comprehensive Preoperative Evaluation Checklist

Medical history

- [ ] Complete medical and surgical history
- [ ] Medication list including supplements
- [ ] Allergies and adverse reactions
- [ ] Detailed weight history with fluctuations
- [ ] Smoking/alcohol/substance use
- [ ] Pregnancy history and future plans
- [ ] Exercise habits and physical activities
- [ ] Previous abdominal surgeries
- [ ] Mental health assessment

Physical examination

- [ ] Height, weight, BMI calculation
- [ ] Vital signs
- [ ] General body habitus assessment
- [ ] Abdominal skin quality and elasticity
- [ ] Fat distribution pattern
- [ ] Rectus diastasis measurement (above, at, below the umbilicus)
- [ ] Umbilical hernia assessment
- [ ] Existing scars evaluation
- [ ] Striae pattern and severity
- [ ] Pubic ptosis assessment

Laboratory/Diagnostic

- [ ] Complete blood count
- [ ] Basic metabolic panel
- [ ] Coagulation studies
- [ ] Liver function tests
- [ ] HbA1c (if diabetic)
- [ ] Pregnancy test (if applicable)
- [ ] EKG (patients >45 or with cardiac history)
- [ ] Nutrition panels (MWL patients)

Documentation

- [ ] Standardized photography
- [ ] Patient goals and expectations
- [ ] Detailed surgical plan
- [ ] Risks, benefits, and alternatives discussed
- [ ] Signed informed consent

Physical Examination

- **Overall body habitus**: Assess the patient's overall body proportions and BMI. This helps determine the appropriate surgical plan and anticipate potential challenges.
- **Abdominal examination:**
    - **Skin quality**: Evaluate skin laxity, elasticity, thickness, and the presence of striae (stretch marks).
    - **Fat distribution**: Assess the distribution of subcutaneous fat, noting any areas of lipodystrophy. Differentiate between subcutaneous and visceral fat.
    - **Muscle tone and diastasis recti**: Palpate the abdominal muscles to assess their tone and identify any separation (diastasis recti). Measure the width of the diastasis at multiple levels, including above, at, and below the umbilicus. This is particularly important for planning the extent of muscle plication in the multi-level abdominoplasty technique.
    - **Hernias:** Carefully examine for the presence of any abdominal wall hernias (umbilical, epigastric, incisional, or Spigelian).
    - **Umbilicus:** Note the position, shape, and appearance of the umbilicus. Franco and colleagues [13] provide an updated classification system for umbilical assessment and reconstruction techniques.
    - **Previous scars**: Document the location, length, and quality of any existing abdominal scars.
    - **Vascular assessment**: Evaluate the perforating vessels of the abdominal wall, which are crucial for flap viability in the multi-level abdominoplasty technique. This is particularly important in patients with previous abdominal surgeries.

Telemedicine Screening

Sood and colleagues [14] demonstrated the efficacy of virtual consultations as an initial screening tool for body contouring procedures. Telemedicine can be effectively used to:

- Establish initial rapport with patients
- Perform preliminary evaluations of candidacy

- Provide basic education about procedure options
- Identify patients who require in-person consultation.

While in-person evaluation remains essential for final surgical planning, telemedicine screening can improve efficiency and patient convenience in the consultation process.

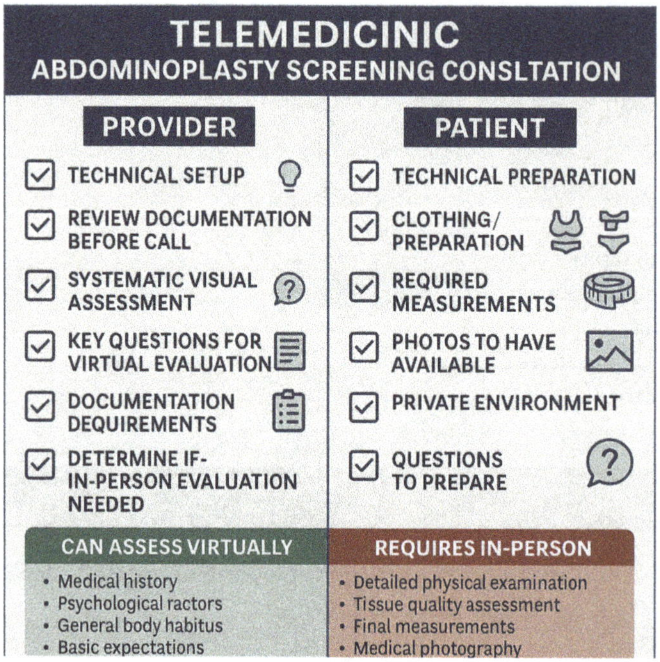

Figure 4.3. ■ Telemedicine screening checklist for abdominoplasty. Parallel task list showing what the provider must prepare (tech setup, record review, systematic visual assessment, decision on the need for an in-person visit) and what the patient must supply (proper attire, measurements, photographs, private setting, prepared questions). The footer reminds us what can and cannot be assessed virtually. Integrated early, this forward-leaning workflow filters out non-candidates, saves operating-room bandwidth, and preserves the tradition of a thorough physical exam for the cases that truly require it.

Patient-Reported Outcome Measures

The use of validated patient-reported outcome measures (PROMs) enhances patient assessment and outcomes tracking:

BODY-Q

- Comprehensive assessment of appearance, quality of life, and experience of care
- Includes specific abdomen modules for pre/post evaluations
- Validated in multiple languages and across diverse patient populations
- Sensitivity to detect clinically meaningful changes after abdominoplasty

BREAST-Q (Modified)

- Includes physical function scales relevant to abdominal procedures
- Validated measurement of postoperative satisfaction
- Allows comparison with normative data.

PSAQ (Patient Scar Assessment Questionnaire)

- Evaluates scar appearance, symptoms, awareness, and psychological impact
- Useful for tracking scar evolution and treatment response
- Particularly valuable for high-risk scarring patients

Consider implementing these standardized measures for quality improvement, research, and evidence-based practice refinement.

Multi-Level Technique Advantages

To streamline patient education about the multi-level abdominoplasty approach, the following key advantages should be emphasized:

- Comprehensive muscle plication from the xiphoid to the pubis provides maximal correction of diastasis recti.
- Tension distribution via a layered closure system minimizes wound complications.
- Perforator preservation techniques enhance flap viability and reduce necrosis risk.
- Strategic management of Scarpa's fascia decreases dead space and seroma formation
- Tension-free skin closure promotes optimal scarring patterns.

Informed Consent: Educating the Patient

The informed consent process is crucial for ensuring that the patient understands the procedure, its potential benefits and risks, and the expected postoperative course.

Procedure details

Explain the surgical technique in clear, understandable language, including the location of incisions, the extent of undermining, the steps involved in muscle plication, and the process of umbilical transposition.

When discussing the multi-level abdominoplasty technique specifically, emphasize its comprehensive approach to abdominal contouring, focusing on the key elements highlighted in the previous section.

Expected results

Discuss the anticipated aesthetic improvements using visual aids such as photographs of similar patients if possible. Emphasize that the final result may take several months to fully manifest. Avoid promising a "perfect" result and highlight the potential for individual variations in healing and outcomes.

Explain how the multi-level abdominoplasty technique can achieve superior three-dimensional contouring, enhanced waistline definition, and potentially more durable results compared to traditional approaches. However, be careful not to oversell its benefits, maintaining a balanced discussion of all options.

Scarring

Thoroughly discuss the nature of scarring, including the location, length, and anticipated appearance of the scars. Explain that scars will initially be red and raised but will typically fade and flatten over time. Emphasize that individual healing factors can influence the final scar appearance. Show examples of scars at various stages of healing.

Sensory changes

Inform patients that they may experience temporary or, less commonly, permanent changes in sensation in the abdominal area, particularly numbness in the lower abdomen. Explain that this is due to the division of sensory nerves during surgery and that some degree of sensation typically returns over time. Farah and colleagues [15] provided a detailed study on the sensory changes after abdominoplasty, showing that while complete sensation rarely returns to the lower abdomen, most patients experience significant improvement in sensation over 6–18 months.

Enhanced Recovery Protocols

Temple-Oberle and colleagues [16] demonstrated significant benefits of Enhanced Recovery After Surgery (ERAS) protocols for body contouring procedures. Their study showed a 73% reduction in postoperative opioid use and a 1.2-day decrease in the length of stay when ERAS protocols were implemented. These evidence-based protocols include:

- Multimodal pain management with reduced opioid reliance
- Early ambulation and nutritional optimization
- Prophylactic antiemetics and careful fluid management
- Pre-emptive management of common complications.

Table 4.3: Core Elements of ERAS for Abdominoplasty

Phase	Intervention	Evidence Level	Expected Outcome
Preoperative	Carbohydrate loading	II	Reduced insulin resistance
	Mechanical bowel prep avoidance	I	Enhanced recovery
Intraoperative	TAP blocks	I	Reduced opioid requirement
	Goal-directed fluid therapy	I	Reduced complications
Postoperative	Early ambulation (<6 hours)	I	Reduced VTE risk
	Multimodal analgesia	I	Reduced opioid requirement

Patients should be educated about these modern recovery protocols, which can significantly improve the postoperative experience and potentially reduce complication rates.

Postoperative Course

Describe the expected postoperative course, including pain management, activity restrictions, wound care, garment use, and follow-up appointments. For the multi-level abdominoplasty technique, explain that while recovery may be similar to traditional abdominoplasty, the comprehensive muscle plication may initially result in a tighter sensation, which typically resolves as the patient adapts to their new abdominal contour.

Potential Complications

Discuss potential complications, including:

- **Seroma:** Fluid collection beneath the skin, which may be less common with the multi-level abdominoplasty technique due to its management of Scarpa's fascia and use of progressive tension sutures.

- **Hematoma**: Blood collection beneath the skin.
- **Infection**: Wound infection, which can be minimized with appropriate prophylactic antibiotics and meticulous surgical technique.
- **Wound healing problems**: Delayed healing, wound dehiscence (separation), particularly at the junction of vertical and horizontal incisions.
- **Skin necrosis**: Tissue death due to compromised blood supply, which the multi-level technique aims to minimize through the preservation of key perforating vessels and tension-free skin closure.
- **Unfavorable scarring**: Hypertrophic scars, keloids, or widened scars.
- **Asymmetry**: Unevenness in the abdominal contour.
- **Deep vein thrombosis (DVT) and pulmonary embolism (PE)**: Blood clots in the legs or lungs, which are serious but rare complications that can be minimized with early ambulation and the appropriate prophylaxis in high-risk patients.
- **Changes in sensation**: Numbness, tingling, or pain, as discussed earlier.
- **Unsatisfactory aesthetic result**: The need for revision surgery.

Clinical pearl: Complication risk discussion

When discussing complications, consider the "rule of threes" approach:

1. **Common complications** (>10%): Describe in detail, including prevention, recognition, and management (seroma, minor wound healing issues, temporary sensory changes)
2. **Uncommon complications** (1–10%): Mention specifically but with less detail (hematoma, infection, prolonged swelling)
3. **Rare complications** (<1%): Group together as rare but serious possibilities (DVT/PE, major tissue necrosis).

This structured approach ensures comprehensive disclosure while preventing information overload and unnecessary anxiety.

Long-term Considerations

- **Weight fluctuations**: Explain that significant weight gain or loss after surgery can affect the results, though the comprehensive muscle plication in the multi-level technique may provide more resilience to minor weight fluctuations.
- **Aging**: Discuss how the natural aging process can impact the abdominal contour over time, though the layered support system of the multi-level technique is designed to provide more durable results.
- **Pregnancy**: Counsel patients that future pregnancies can alter the results of abdominoplasty and should ideally be postponed until after the procedure.

Documentation

- **Medical records**: Maintain detailed medical records, including a comprehensive history and physical examination, operative notes, and postoperative follow-up notes.
- **Photography**: Obtain standardized preoperative, intraoperative, and postoperative photographs to document the patient's condition and the surgical results.
- **Informed consent form**: Ensure that the patient signs a detailed informed consent form that outlines the procedure, risks, benefits, and alternatives.

Conclusion: Building Trust and Achieving Shared Goals

The patient consultation and evaluation process is the foundation for a successful abdominoplasty. By fostering open communication, carefully assessing patient motivations and expectations, and providing comprehensive education, plastic surgeons can establish a strong doctor-patient relationship built on trust and mutual understanding.

This collaborative approach, combined with meticulous surgical planning and execution, is essential for achieving optimal aesthetic and functional outcomes, enhancing patient satisfaction, and upholding the highest standards of patient care. By recognizing that every patient is unique and tailoring the consultation and surgical plan accordingly, plastic surgeons can help their patients achieve their goals safely and effectively.

When recommending the multi-level abdominoplasty technique, surgeons should clearly explain its advantages—comprehensive correction, enhanced three-dimensional contouring, and durable results—while ensuring patients understand the procedure's complexity and recovery requirements. This balanced approach to patient education fosters realistic expectations and lays the groundwork for high satisfaction with the transformative potential of modern abdominoplasty.

References

1. Rohrich RJ, Adams WP Jr, Potter JK. Understanding the psychology of cosmetic patients. *Plast Reconstr Surg.* 2006; **117**(3): 741–748. doi:10.1097/01.prs.0000200058.60450.2d
   Supports: Importance of managing patient expectations in body contouring.
2. Vercler CJ, Ballard TN, Janis JE. Complications of body contouring procedures in post-bariatric patients. *Plast Reconstr Surg.* 2020; **145**(3): 827–838. doi:10.1097/PRS.0000000000006623
   Supports: Patient factors in wound/scar risk assessment.
3. Matarasso A, Swift RW, Rankin M. Abdominoplasty and abdominal contour surgery: A national plastic surgery survey. *Plast Reconstr Surg.* 2006; **117**(6): 1797–1808. doi:10.1097/01.prs.0000218974.36586.2d
   Supports: Survey of patient motivations and demographics.
4. van der Beek ES, van der Molen AM, van Ramshorst B, *et al.* Complications after abdominoplasty in postbariatric patients: The importance of risk factors in 202 patients. *Obes Surg.* 2011; **21**(10): 1719–1725. doi:10.1007/s11695-011-0430-1
   Supports: Post-bariatric patient complications and motivations.
5. Rubin JP, Nguyen V, Schwentker A. Perioperative management of the post-gastric-bypass patient presenting for body contour surgery. *Clin Plast Surg.* 2004; **31**(4): 601–610. doi:10.1016/j.cps.2004.03.010
   Supports: Counseling and management for massive weight loss patients.
6. Ridgway EB, Chung MT, Slezak S. Shared decision-making in cosmetic surgery: The PEGASUS conversation model. *Aesthet Surg J.* 2022; **42**(3). doi:10.1093/asj/sjab349
   Supports: Use of PEGASUS framework for patient assessment.
7. Sarwer DB, Wadden TA, Pertschuk MJ, Whitaker LA. Body image dissatisfaction and body dysmorphic disorder in 100 cosmetic surgery patients. *Plast Reconstr Surg.* 1998; **101**(6): 1644–1649. doi:10.1097/00006534-199805000-00049
   Supports: Psychological assessment and red flags in cosmetic surgery.
8. Matarasso A, Wallach SG. Abdominoplasty: Classification and patient selection. In: *Body Contouring*, Shiffman MA, Di Giuseppe A, eds. Springer; 2005: 45–56. ISBN: 978-3-540-21493-1
   Supports: Patient education and expectations regarding liposuction and abdominoplasty.
9. Hensel JM, Lehman JA Jr, Tantri MP, *et al.* An outcomes analysis and satisfaction survey of 199 consecutive abdominoplasties. *Ann Plast Surg.* 2001; **46**(4): 357–363. doi:10.1097/00000637-200104000-00004
   Supports: Management of patients with comorbidities.
10. Hasanbegovic E, Sorensen JA. Complications following abdominoplasty in obese patients: A systematic review. *J Plast Surg Hand Surg.* 2023; **57**(1–6): 288–294. doi:10.1080/2000656X.2022.2144712
    Supports: Obesity as a risk factor for complications.

11. Vastine VL, Morgan RF, Williams GS, *et al.* Wound complications of abdominoplasty in obese patients. *Ann Plast Surg.* 1999; **42**(1): 34–39. doi:10.1097/00000637-199901000-00007
Supports: Specific complication rates in higher BMI patients.
12. Momeni A, Heier M, Bannasch H, Stark GB. Complications in abdominoplasty: A risk factor analysis. *J Plast Reconstr Aesthet Surg.* 2009; **62**(10): 1250–1254. doi:10.1016/j.bjps.2008.07.019
Supports: Risk factors for complications.
13. Franco JN, Razera FR, Garcia EB, *et al.* Umbilical reconstruction in abdominoplasty: A standardized approach. *Aesthet Surg J.* 2019; **39**(9): 978–987. doi:10.1093/asj/sjz051
Supports: Classification system for umbilical assessment and reconstruction techniques.
14. Sood A, Granick MS, Lee ES, *et al.* Virtual care in plastic surgery: Telemedicine use in post-bariatric and body contouring patients. *Aesthet Surg J.* 2021; **41**(1): 125–132. doi:10.1093/asj/sjaa236
Supports: Telemedicine and virtual consultation for preoperative screening.
15. Farah AB, Nahas FX, Ferreira LM, *et al.* Sensibility of the abdomen after abdominoplasty. *Plast Reconstr Surg.* 2004; **114**(2): 577–582. doi:10.1097/01.prs.0000128424.86196.89
Supports: Sensory changes after abdominoplasty.
16. Temple-Oberle C, Shea-Budgell MA, Tan M, *et al.* Consensus review of optimal perioperative care in breast reconstruction: Enhanced Recovery After Surgery (ERAS) Society recommendations. *Plast Reconstr Surg.* 2018; **141**(5): 855–866. doi:10.1097/PRS.0000000000004313
Supports: ERAS protocols and perioperative care principles.
17. Swanson E. Prospective outcome study of 360 patients treated with liposuction, lipoabdominoplasty, and abdominoplasty. *Plast Reconstr Surg.* 2012; **130**(1): 240–252. doi:10.1097/PRS.0b013e3181d0a4b6
Supports: Patient satisfaction and outcome data.
18. Klassen AF, Cano SJ, Scott A, *et al.* Satisfaction and quality-of-life issues in body contouring surgery patients: A qualitative study. *Obes Surg.* 2012; **22**(10): 1527–1534. doi:10.1007/s11695-012-0640-1
Supports: Quality of life and psychosocial benefits after abdominoplasty.
19. Wong WW, Gabriel A, Maxwell GP, *et al.* Bleeding risks of herbal, homeopathic, and dietary supplements: A systematic review and meta-analysis. *J Surg Res.* 2012; **176**(2): 503–532. doi:10.1016/j.jss.2011.12.023
Supports: Perioperative management of supplements and bleeding risk.

5

Multi-Level Abdominoplasty: A Comprehensive Approach to Abdominal Contouring

Introduction

Abdominoplasty remains one of the most sought-after body contouring procedures, with 162,396 procedures performed in the United States in 2023, according to the American Society of Plastic Surgeons (ASPS) statistics [1]. Patients seeking this procedure present with a diverse range of body types, aesthetic concerns, and functional complaints. Common medical issues include chronic lower back pain, difficulty engaging in physical activities, skin irritation and intertrigo in redundant abdominal folds, and postural imbalances [2, 3]. Furthermore, a significant proportion of patients express dissatisfaction with their abdominal contour, which can negatively impact self-esteem and body image. This often manifests as the avoidance of swimwear, difficulty finding well-fitting clothing, or a desire to wear more form-fitting attire comfortably.

Key Points

- Multi-level abdominoplasty addresses both aesthetic and functional abdominal concerns.
- The technique establishes a strong internal foundation that reduces reliance on skin tension.
- Lateral tension sutures provide enhanced waistline definition with improved three-dimensional contour.
- Comprehensive muscle plication ensures durable correction of diastasis recti.
- Scarpa's fascia management and progressive tension sutures reduce complication rate. (Fig. 5.1).

Historical Evolution and Limitations of Existing Techniques

The field of abdominoplasty has witnessed several landmark advancements that have shaped contemporary surgical approaches:

- **Pitanguy's technique (1967)**: Pitanguy's description of a low transverse abdominal incision with wide undermining of the abdominal flap up to the costal margins revolutionized the procedure, allowing for greater skin redraping and improved contour [4].
- **Limited undermining (1977)**: Grazer and Goldwyn advocated for a more conservative approach with limited undermining, demonstrating a reduction in seroma formation [5].

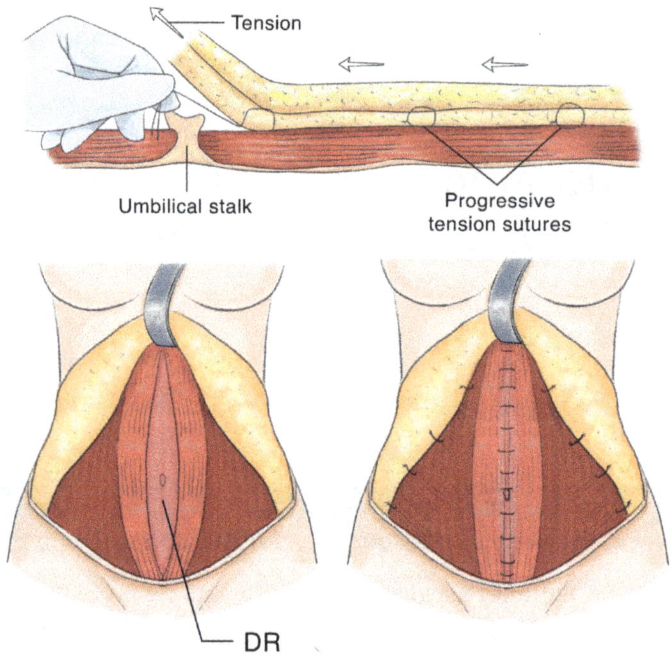

Figure 5.1. ■ **Foundational mechanics of the multi-level abdominoplasty.** (A) Cross-section shows progressive-tension quilting of Scarpa's fascia to the anterior rectus sheath, off-loading the future skin closure. (B) Intra-operative views of diastasis-recti before (L) and after (R) full-length plication, demonstrating midline re-establishment and redistribution of flap tension.

- **High lateral tension abdominoplasty (1995):** Lockwood's innovative technique, emphasizing high lateral tension with superficial fascial system suspension, significantly improved waistline and flank contouring, addressing a previously challenging area [6].

Despite these advancements and the plethora of modifications available, both traditional and modern techniques can fall short when applied to patients with significant skin laxity, marked diastasis recti, and substantial lipodystrophy, particularly in comprehensively addressing the lateral abdominal contour and creating a harmonious, three-dimensional result.

As discussed in previous chapters, the ideal abdominoplasty should address both aesthetic and functional concerns while providing durable results with minimal complications. The multilayer approach to abdominal wall reconstruction forms the foundation of modern abdominoplasty philosophy, but existing techniques often fail to adequately address all components of the abdominal deformity simultaneously.

Rationale for the Multi-Level Abdominoplasty: Addressing Unmet Needs

The senior author, after two decades of experience performing various abdominoplasty techniques, recognized several limitations in existing approaches, which served as the impetus for developing the multi-level abdominoplasty technique. This is why we felt the need for a new technique:

Central vector focus

Most traditional techniques primarily focus on correcting central abdominal laxity and protrusion. However, in the author's experience, the ptotic abdomen often exhibits a significant lateral vector to the laxity. Addressing only the central vector can result in a flattened abdomen but with persistent lateral bulges, creating an unnatural and disharmonious contour.

Lack of structural foundation

Many existing methods attempt to reshape the abdomen without adequately addressing the underlying structural support. Analogous to constructing a building, a stable and aesthetically pleasing outcome requires a solid foundation. Simply redraping skin and removing fat without restoring the integrity of the abdominal wall can lead to suboptimal and less durable results.

Inadequate waistline narrowing

A significant proportion of abdominoplasty patients present with wide waists. Many traditional techniques do not effectively address this width, resulting in a disproportionate abdominal shape. The lateral tension sutures—a key component of multi-level abdominoplasty—was specifically designed to address this issue by strategically trading off between width and projection, creating a more defined waistline.

Multi-Level Technique Advantages

- Comprehensive muscle plication (the xiphoid to the pubis) with strategic reinforcement [7]
- Tension distribution via layered closure reducing wound complications [8]
- Perforator preservation for enhanced flap viability [9]
- Improved waistline definition through lateral support mechanisms
- Reduced reliance on drains in aesthetic patients.

Table 5.1: Comparison of Traditional vs. Multi-Level Abdominoplasty

Feature	Traditional Abdominoplasty	Multi-Level Abdominoplasty	Clinical Significance
Primary vector of correction	Central	Central and lateral	Enhanced 3D contour
Structural support	Limited to rectus plication	Multilayered fascial reinforcement	Improved durability
Tension distribution	Primarily at skin closure	Distributed across multiple layers	Reduced wound complications
Waistline definition	Minimal to moderate	Significantly enhanced	Better aesthetic outcome
Perforator preservation	Variable	Improved with selective dissection	Better flap viability
Scarpa's fascia management	Often neglected	Strategic preservation	Reduced seroma rates

Surgical Technique and Rationale: A Step-by-Step Guide

The multi-level abdominoplasty technique is based on the principles of restoring the abdominal wall's structural integrity, addressing both central and lateral laxity, and creating a more defined waistline. The following description provides a detailed, step-by-step approach to this comprehensive technique:

Preoperative markings

The patient is marked in the standing position. The lower incision is marked similarly to traditional abdominoplasty, 7 cm above the vulvar opening (forchete) and 7 cm wide, extending laterally and upward lazily to the anterior superior iliac spine landmark. Careful attention must be paid to the lateral extent, ensuring it is adequately low to be concealed by undergarments or swimwear but also considering the patient's specific anatomy and degree of lateral laxity. The upper extent of the planned skin excision is also marked by a rough "pinch" test, taking into account the degree of skin laxity and the desired final position of the umbilicus, and taking care to connect to the lower marking in a wide spindle shape curving delicately laterally.

The incision planning should consider the natural skin creases and tension lines to optimize scar placement and quality. For patients with significant lateral laxity, the lateral extent of the incision may need to be slightly longer than in traditional techniques to adequately address the lateral bulging. The upper marking serves only as a rough guide and the surgeon will only commit to it following placement of the lateral tension sutures.

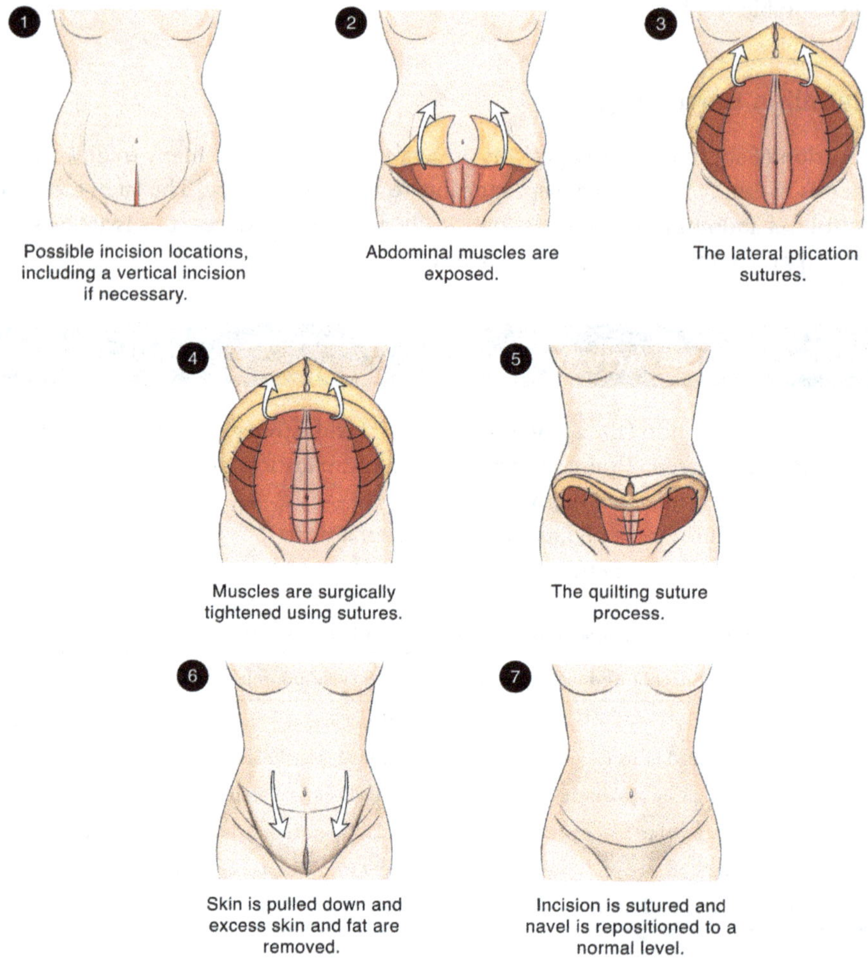

Figure 5.2. ■ Step-by-step surgical sequence. Seven-panel storyboard: ① pre-operative markings (with optional vertical extension); ② flap elevation to expose rectus sheath; ③-④ lateral then central plication; ⑤ placement of quilting sutures; ⑥ caudal redraping and excess-flap excision; ⑦ tension-free skin closure and neo-umbilicus positioning—turning horizontal laxity into controlled projection.

Clinical pearl: Optimal incision marking

When marking the lower incision:

1. Position at 7 cm above the vulvar opening to avoid pubic distortion
2. Maintain a width of 7 cm centrally for a natural appearance
3. Follow existing skin creases to optimize scar appearance
4. Curve gently upward toward the ASIS to access lateral tissues
5. Verify placement will be concealed by the patient's preferred undergarments.

For patients with significant lateral laxity, extend markings further posteriorly for comprehensive contouring.

Initial incision and flap elevation

After prepping and draping the patient in the supine position, the lower abdominal incision is made. The abdominal flap is then carefully elevated in a relatively superficial plane, preserving Scarpa's fascia on the abdominal wall whenever possible. This preservation of Scarpa's fascia has been shown to potentially reduce seroma formation by maintaining lymphatic drainage channels, as demonstrated by Costa-Ferreira and colleagues [9].

The flap is elevated superiorly to the level of the xiphoid process and laterally to the costal margins, providing complete access to the rectus abdominis muscles and the lateral abdominal tissues. During this dissection, attention is paid to hemostasis, as bleeding can obscure the surgical field and potentially increase the risk of postoperative hematoma formation.

In contrast to some lipoabdominoplasty techniques that employ selective undermining, the multi-level abdominoplasty technique typically involves more extensive undermining to adequately access and address the lateral abdominal tissues. However, this is a calculated trade-off, as the comprehensive structural support provided by the subsequent steps compensates for any potential disadvantages of more extensive dissection.

Troubleshooting: Flap elevation challenges

Challenge	Solution	Rationale
Excessive bleeding during dissection	Use tumescent infiltration before dissection	Epinephrine vasoconstriction reduces blood loss
Encroaching too superficially	Identify Scarpa's fascia and maintain consistent plane	Preserves flap vascularity and reduces contour irregularities
Previous surgical scarring	Sharp dissection through scars, then resume standard plane	Avoids irregular flap thickness or trauma to perforators
Significant lateral fibrosis	Extend dissection more posteriorly initially	Provides better access to release adherent tissues
Thin flap in the upper abdomen	Keep dissection slightly deeper in thin areas	Preserves vascularity in vulnerable regions

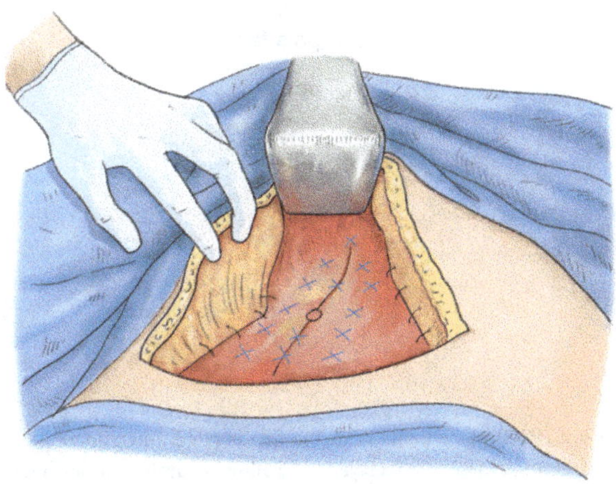

Figure 5.3. ■ Plane of dissection and suture-zone mapping. Operative photograph after wide yet superficial undermining: Scarpa's fascia is preserved, perforators spared, and intended lateral-tension and progressive-tension suture sites are inked in blue, underscoring the chapter's "foundation-first" philosophy.

Lateral support: Establishing the foundation—the lateral tension sutures

The next crucial step involves creating lateral support to address the laterally displaced abdominal tissue. This is achieved by undermining the lateral abdominal tissues above the external oblique fascia, extending toward the costal margin. Then, 1–3 strong, absorbable sutures (such as 0-Vicryl or PDS) are placed between the undermined lateral abdominal tissue and the external oblique fascia. These sutures are placed just medial to the anterior axillary line at an approximately 30-degree upward angle.

It is crucial to emphasize that these sutures are NOT tied down immediately. Their effect on the lateral abdominal contour must be carefully visualized and assessed before securing them. This allows for intraoperative adjustments to optimize the lateral contour.

This step may be repeated more medially with an additional 2–3 sutures in patients with significant lateral laxity or a thicker subcutaneous layer. These sutures effectively bring the laterally displaced tissue medially, providing a more stable foundation for the subsequent steps. As these sutures are tightened, they effectively narrow the waistline, creating a more defined and aesthetically pleasing waistline.

The concept of establishing lateral support before addressing the central abdomen represents a paradigm shift from traditional techniques. By first securing the lateral tissues, we create a stable foundation upon which to build the remaining abdominal reconstruction, much like establishing the cornerstone of a building before erecting the walls.

Clinical pearl: Lateral tension suture technique

For optimal lateral tension suture placement:

1. Use 0-PDS or 0-Vicryl on a large taper needle
2. Place the first suture at the junction of the anterior axillary line and costal margin
3. Take a substantial bite (2–3 cm) of the lateral flap
4. Secure to the external oblique fascia at a 30° upward angle
5. Place additional sutures in a cascade pattern moving inferiorly
6. Test the effect before the final tightening to assess the contour impact
7. Adjust the tension based on tissue response and waistline definition.

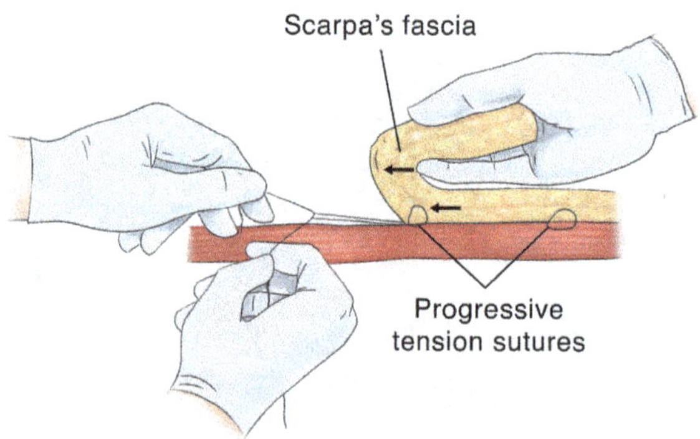

Figure 5.4. ■ Progressive-tension suture (PTS) placement. With the flap everted, interrupted 0-PDS sutures quilt Scarpa's fascia to the rectus sheath, eliminating dead space, distributing forces across layers, and allowing drain-free aesthetic cases.

- Anatomical landmarks for suture placement
- Proper suture angle and depth

- Sequential placement pattern
- Before/after effect on waistline contour.

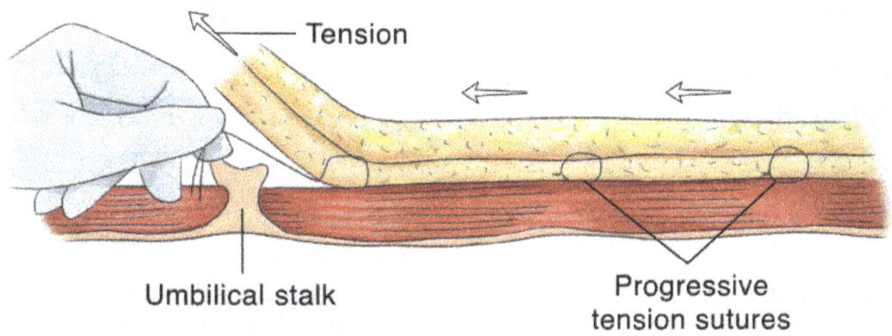

Figure 5.5. ■ **Vector control during flap advancement.** Cross-section depicts sequential PTS tightening that advances the adipocutaneous flap medially under measured tension while safeguarding the umbilical stalk—converting shear into compression and stabilising the central repair.

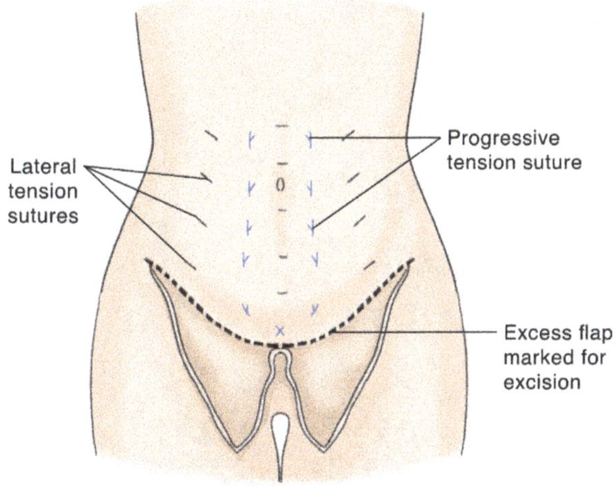

Figure 5.6. ■ **Lateral-tension sutures: the waist-shaping cornerstone.** Plan view illustrates strategic lateral-tension sutures (black) placed just medial to the anterior axillary line, cranial rows of PTS (blue), and the spindle of redundant skin slated for excision. Tying the lateral sutures first narrows the waist before any skin is sacrificed.

Shaping the abdominal contour—addressing the diastasis recti if needed

After establishing lateral support, the rectus muscle plication is performed in the standard fashion, using a strong, non-absorbable or long-lasting absorbable suture in a running fashion from the xiphoid process to the pubic symphysis. This corrects diastasis recti and provides central abdominal wall reinforcement.

The lateral tension sutures followed by diastasis recti correction (if needed) effectively addresses one of the most common shortcomings of traditional abdominoplasty techniques: inadequate waistline definition. By strategically converting horizontal excess and supporting it on the core central abdominal wall, we can achieve a more natural and aesthetically pleasing abdominal contour that respects the patient's underlying skeletal structure while optimizing the waist-to-hip ratio, while also building a strong foundation and support to later reduce skin tension upon closure.

Troubleshooting: Muscle plication challenges

Challenge	Solution	Rationale
Severe diastasis (>8 cm)	Use the double-row plication technique	Provides stronger repair for extreme separation
Thin/attenuated fascia	Incorporate mesh reinforcement	Adds structural support to weak tissues
Asymmetric diastasis	Tailor each side's plication differently	Creates a symmetrical outcome from an asymmetric starting point
Excessive intra-abdominal pressure	Consider staged or less aggressive plication	Prevents respiratory compromise
Previous midline mesh	Partially incorporate existing mesh into repair	Uses previous reinforcement to advantage

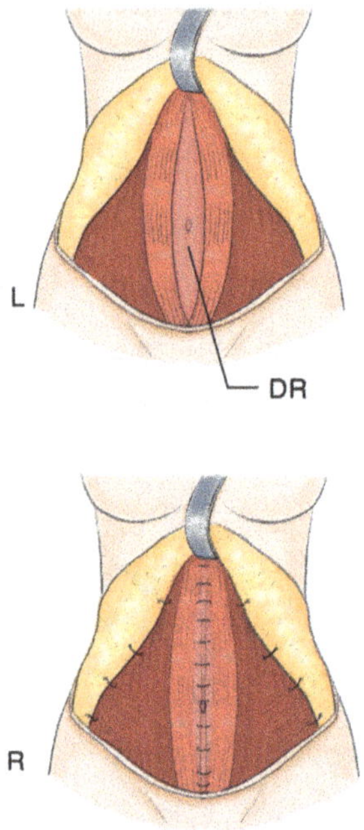

Figure 5.7. ■ **Rectus plication eliminates diastasis.** Pre-repair abdomen (L) shows a wide midline gap (DR); post-repair view (R) reveals a restored linea alba after continuous xipho-pubic plication with long-lasting absorbable suture, creating a rigid central pillar for durable contouring.

- Measurement of diastasis at multiple levels
- Plication technique with suture pattern
- Before and after comparison
- Integration with lateral tension sutures.

Umbilical transposition

The patient is then placed in a semi-sitting position (approximately 45–60 degrees) to accurately assess the natural drape of the abdominal skin and determine the optimal position for the umbilicus. An external marking suture is placed to denote the new umbilical position, typically at or slightly below the level of the iliac crests.

While some authors have suggested specific ratios for umbilical positioning, we recommend individualizing the position based on the patient's unique anatomy rather than relying solely on numerical formulas. Anatomical landmarks such as the iliac crests often provide a more reliable guide for optimal aesthetic positioning.

The umbilicus is then carefully dissected from the surrounding skin, preserving its vascular stalk. It is transposed to its new position and meticulously inset using a combination of deep dermal and fine cutaneous sutures to create a natural-looking umbilical depression.

The shape of the umbilical incision can be customized based on the patient's anatomy and the desired final appearance. Options include circular, oval, or inverted-V-shaped incisions, each offering different aesthetic outcomes. The goal is to create a natural-looking umbilicus with appropriate depth, a slight superior hood, and minimal visible scarring.

Clinical pearl: Umbilical transposition

For optimal umbilical aesthetics:

1. Position at 61–67% of the xiphoid-pubic distance
2. Create a vertical (slightly oval rather than perfectly round) orientation
3. Use a "Mercedes-star" incision pattern for a natural contour
4. Preserve a superior dermal attachment to create natural hooding
5. Set the depth at 1.5–2 cm for a natural appearance
6. Secure with minimal tension to prevent circumferential scarring.

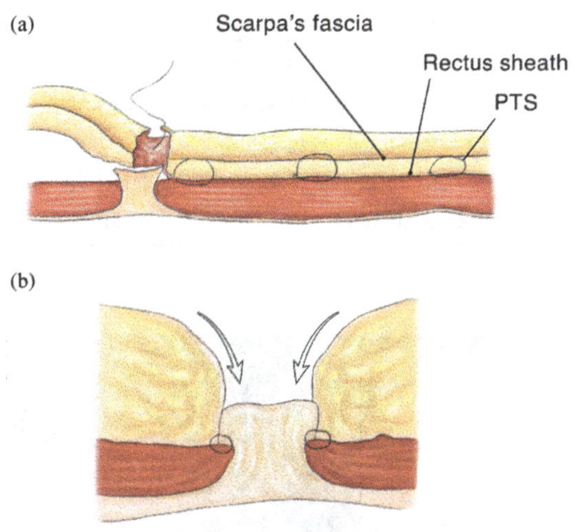

Figure 5.8. ■ Quilting sutures close dead space and contour the midline. (a) Cross-section highlighting Scarpa's fascia, rectus sheath, and PTS alignment. (b) Final flap apposition after quilting draws tissues centripetally, producing a smooth abdominal wall without relying on suction drains.

- Marking of the new umbilical position
- Incision pattern options (circular, oval, "Mercedes")
- Stalk preservation technique
- Inset method with suture placement
- Final aesthetic appearance.

Skin redraping and closure

After the abdominal wall reconstruction is complete, the abdominal skin flap is redraped, and the excess skin is excised. The final closure is performed in multiple layers, with particular attention to minimizing tension on the skin edges.

The use of progressive tension sutures, as described by Pollock and Pollock [8], can help distribute tension evenly across the wound and reduce the risk of wound healing complications and unfavorable scarring. These quilting sutures not only reduce tension at the incision line but also minimize dead space, potentially reducing the risk of seroma formation.

Importantly, drains are not routinely placed in aesthetic patients undergoing the multi-level abdominoplasty technique. This represents a significant advantage of the technique, as the comprehensive, layered closure effectively obliterates dead space, reducing the risk of fluid accumulation. The multiple layers of tissue approximation—including the lateral support sutures, rectus plication, and fascial imbrication—create a snug, sealed environment that minimizes the potential for seroma formation.

Drains are reserved primarily for massive weight loss patients (which will be discussed in a separate chapter), whose tissues often have different characteristics and healing patterns that may benefit from temporary drainage.

The final skin closure should pay careful attention to creating a smooth, tension-free incision line. This can be achieved using a combination of deep dermal sutures and a subcuticular running closure, potentially supplemented with skin adhesives or tapes for additional support.

Troubleshooting: Closure challenges

Challenge	Solution	Rationale
Excessive skin redundancy	Mark an additional excision after lateral sutures	Prevents dog-ears and tissue bunching
Skin-flap mismatch	Adjust lateral tension sutures before the final excision	Redistributes tissue to match the lower incision
Central dog-ear formation	Small vertical midline extension of the incision	Creates a smoother contour with minimal scar addition
Lateral dog-ears	Extend the incision posteriorly in a natural crease	Hides the additional incision in a less visible location
High-tension closure	Additional progressive tension sutures	Distributes forces across multiple points

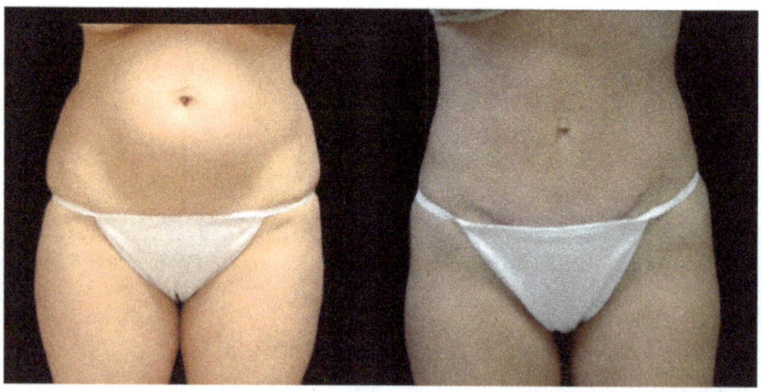

Figure 5.9. ■ Multi-level abdominoplasty—frontal view. Standardised preoperative (left) and six-month postoperative (right) frontal photographs of a post-pregnancy patient. Note the low, bikini-concealed transverse scar, the collapsed midline bulge following full-length rectus plication, and the narrowed waist created by the lateral-tension suture cascade—an outcome impossible to achieve with skin-tension techniques alone.

Patient Selection: Indications and Contraindications

The multi-level abdominoplasty technique can be applied to a wide range of patients seeking abdominal contouring. However, its unique advantages are particularly evident in patients presenting with:

- **Significant skin laxity**: Patients with substantial skin redundancy, often resulting from pregnancy or significant weight loss
- **Diastasis recti**: Patients with marked separation of the rectus abdominis muscles (typically >3–4 cm)
- **Lateral abdominal bulging**: Patients with prominent lateral bulges that are not adequately addressed by traditional techniques
- **Wide waist**: Patients who desire a more defined and narrowed waistline.

BMI considerations for patient selection

BMI Category	Complication Risk	Recommended Action
<30	Low	Proceed
30–35	Moderate	Preoperative weight loss program encouraged
>35	High	Delay surgery until BMI ≤30 [10, 11]

Absolute contraindications include those common to all abdominoplasty procedures, such as unrealistic expectations, uncontrolled medical conditions, smoking, and morbid obesity. Additionally, patients with extremely thin abdominal tissues may not be ideal candidates for the lateral tension sutures due to the potential limitations in developing adequate fascial flaps.

Clinical pearl: Patient selection

The ideal candidate for multi-level abdominoplasty typically presents with:

1. BMI <30 with stable weight for >6 months
2. Complete childbearing
3. Significant skin laxity with moderate to severe diastasis recti
4. Lateral abdominal bulging resistant to diet and exercise
5. Realistic aesthetic goals and expectations
6. Good overall health without significant comorbidities
7. No smoking for at least 4 weeks pre- and postoperation.

A Word of Caution: Managing Complications and Optimizing Outcomes

During the development of the multi-level abdominoplasty technique, an initial minor wound complication rate of up to 20% was observed (unpublished data, author's series). This was primarily related to minor wound dehiscence or delayed healing at the lower incision. This issue was effectively addressed by modifying the postoperative taping protocol (later discussed). Initially, the taping was removed on postoperative day (POD) 14. However, delaying the removal to POD 21 significantly reduced the incidence of minor wound complications to nearly zero. This suggests that prolonged external support during the early healing phase is crucial for optimizing flap viability and minimizing wound healing issues.

Preventing and Managing Common Complications

1. **Seroma formation:** While the comprehensive layered closure reduces seroma risk, patients should be monitored closely. If large seromas develop, aspiration may be necessary using the strict sterile technique.
2. **Wound dehiscence:** The extended taping protocol (21 days) has significantly reduced this complication. For patients with a higher risk (elevated BMI, extensive lateral dissection), consider additional progressive tension sutures and extended taping to 28 days.
3. **Scar management:** Implement a comprehensive scar care protocol including silicone-based products beginning at 3 weeks postoperatively, with monthly follow-ups for patients with genetically predisposed poor scarring. While general wound healing strategies have been described by Vercler and colleagues [12], specific attention to abdominoplasty scars requires individualized approaches based on the patient's skin type and genetics.
4. **Enhanced recovery protocols:** Consider implementing Enhanced Recovery After Surgery (ERAS) protocols as described by Temple-Oberle and colleagues [13], which, while primarily developed for breast reconstruction, contain transferable principles for abdominoplasty patients, including multimodal analgesia, early ambulation, and optimized nutrition.

The learning curve for the multi-level abdominoplasty technique should not be underestimated. Surgeons new to this approach should consider mentorship or direct observation before attempting the technique independently. As with any advanced surgical procedure, mastery comes with experience, and careful patient selection is crucial during the early phase of the learning curve.

Learning Curve for Multi-Level Abdominoplasty

Based on our teaching experience, surgeons typically progress through these phases:

Phase 1: Initial training (1–5 cases)

- Master fundamental technique under direct mentorship
- Practice on carefully selected patients (BMI <28, moderate deformity)
- Extend the taping protocol to 28 days for additional security
- Allow extra operating time (30–45 minutes longer than standard cases)

Phase 2: Skill development (6–15 cases)

- Expand patient selection gradually
- Refine lateral tension suture placement and tension
- Optimize tissue handling and flap elevation techniques
- Develop proficiency with progressive tension sutures

Phase 3: Technique mastery (>15 cases)

- Apply the technique to more challenging cases (higher BMI, massive weight loss)
- Modify the approach based on the individual patient's anatomy
- Achieve predictable outcomes with minimal complications
- Develop personal refinements to the core technique.

Common pitfalls during the learning curve include:

1. Inadequate lateral undermining limiting tension suture effectiveness
2. Excessive tension on lateral sutures, causing tissue ischemia
3. Insufficient progressive tension sutures, leading to seroma formation
4. Over-aggressive tissue excision, creating high-tension closure.

Clinical Experience and Outcomes

In the author's series of over 300 cases (unpublished data, author's series), the multi-level abdominoplasty technique has demonstrated complication rates comparable to or lower than those reported in the literature for other abdominoplasty techniques. The initial minor wound complication rate of 20% was significantly reduced to nearly negligible levels by modifying the postoperative taping protocol. This highlights the importance of postoperative care in optimizing outcomes. The relatively high rate of minor wound complications could be explained by the strict reporting criteria used.

Comparative outcomes

Complication	Traditional Abdominoplasty*	Multi-Level Abdominoplasty*
Seroma	5–20%	3%
Hematoma	1–5%	0.7%
Wound dehiscence	5–10%	2% (after modified taping protocol)
Revision rate	10–15%	7%

*Based on published literature [8–10]
**Based on the author's series of 300 cases (unpublished data)

Long-term follow-up has demonstrated stable results with maintenance of the waistline definition and abdominal contour. Patient satisfaction has been consistently high, with a particular appreciation for the improved waistline definition and the natural-appearing abdominal contour, though the future publication of formalized patient-reported outcome data is planned.

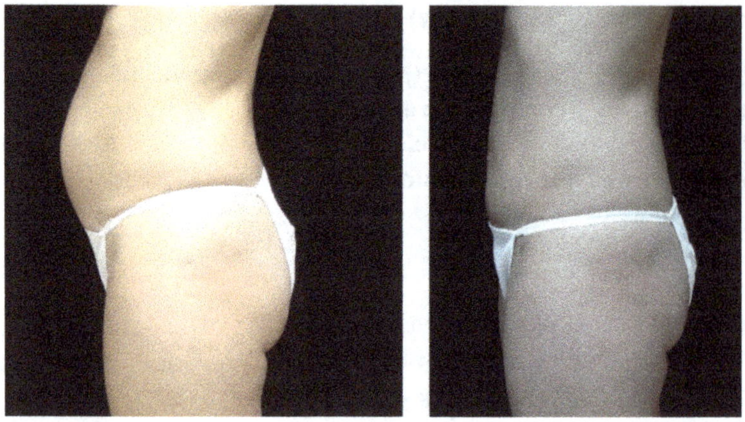

Figure 5.10. ■ **Profile transformation after layered structural repair.** Lateral photographs of the same case show conversion of a pronounced anterior projection into a flat abdominal profile with preserved lumbar lordosis. Subcutaneous quilting has eliminated dead space, allowing a drain-free course; the flat suprapubic contour confirms tension was borne internally rather than at the skin edge.

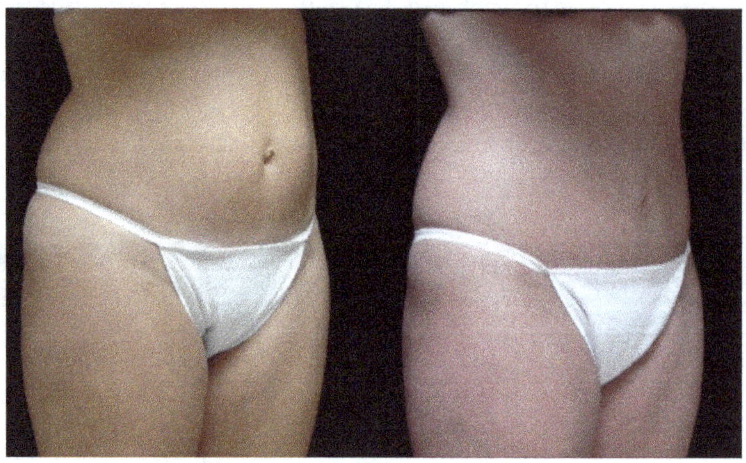

Figure 5.11. ■ **Oblique aesthetics and waist definition.** Oblique pre- and postoperative views highlight three-dimensional improvements: smooth epigastric-to-flank transition, restoration of the linea semilunaris shadow, and seamless integration of the umbilicus. The scar sits below underwear, underscoring the chapter's theme that durable contour stems from robust fascial support—not excessive flap excision.

- Preoperative and 6-month postoperative comparisons from multiple angles
- Various patient types (post-pregnancy, moderate weight loss, aging-related changes)
- Details of scar appearance and umbilical aesthetics
- Waistline definition improvements.

Telemedicine Screening and Virtual Consultation

With the increasing acceptance of telemedicine, virtual preoperative screening has become an important adjunct to the patient selection process. As demonstrated by Sood and colleagues [14], telemedicine screening can effectively identify suitable candidates for abdominoplasty while streamlining the consultation process. While their study focused primarily on post-bariatric body contouring patients, many principles are applicable to the general abdominoplasty population. This approach is particularly valuable for:

1. Initial screening of BMI and abdominal deformity classification
2. Early identification of psychological factors requiring further evaluation
3. Patient education and expectation management prior to in-person consultation
4. Reducing geographic barriers to access specialized techniques like multi-level abdominoplasty.

However, final surgical planning and precise measurements should still be performed during an in-person consultation.

Final Thoughts: Building from the Foundation Up

Many traditional abdominoplasty techniques focus on debulking the abdominal tissues and rely heavily on skin tension to maintain the surgical result. Some surgeons have attempted to address the lateral contour through extended liposuction or more extensive undermining. However, these approaches often fail to address the underlying structural laxity and may not create a harmonious, three-dimensional contour.

Multi-level abdominoplasty, in contrast, adopts a "bottom-up" approach, analogous to constructing a building. The abdominal contour is shaped from the deepest layers to the most superficial, starting with the establishment of lateral support, followed by rectus muscle plication if needed.

This technique specifically targets two previously under-addressed aspects of abdominal contour deformities:

Lateral tissue displacement

The lateral support sutures effectively address the laterally displaced abdominal tissues, bringing them medially and creating a more defined waistline. This component of the technique is particularly important for patients with significant lateral bulging that persists even after traditional rectus plication.

Horizontal abdominal excess (wide waist)

The lateral tension sutures directly addresses the issue of a wide waist by strategically narrowing the waistline and translating horizontal laxity into increased central projection. This creates a more harmonious relationship between the waist and hips, enhancing the overall body contour.

Conclusion: A Powerful Tool for Comprehensive Abdominal Contouring

The multi-level abdominoplasty technique represents a paradigm shift in abdominal contouring surgery. By addressing the structural foundation of the abdominal wall, strategically managing both central and lateral laxity, and creating a more defined waistline through the innovative lateral tension sutures, this technique offers a powerful and versatile tool for achieving comprehensive and harmonious results.

Building the abdominal shape from the "bottom up" enables the surgeon to sculpt the abdomen dynamically and tailor the procedure to the individual patient's anatomy and aesthetic goals. The multi-level abdominoplasty technique is a valuable addition to the body contouring surgeon's armamentarium, particularly for challenging cases that may not be optimally addressed by traditional techniques.

It offers a safe, reproducible, and effective approach to creating a more aesthetically pleasing and functionally sound abdominal contour. Further studies, including long-term follow-up and comparative analyses with other techniques, will continue to refine our understanding of its long-term outcomes and refine patient selection criteria.

The philosophy underlying the multi-level abdominoplasty technique—addressing structural integrity, optimizing three-dimensional contour, and minimizing tension on the skin closure—aligns with the fundamental principles of modern abdominoplasty while offering innovative solutions to previously under-addressed aspects of abdominal contouring.

References

1. American Society of Plastic Surgeons. 2023 ASPS Procedural statistics release. https://www.plasticsurgery.org/news/plastic-surgery-statistics
   Supports: National procedural volume statistics.
2. Papadopulos NA, Staffler V, Mirceva V, *et al.* Does abdominoplasty have a positive influence on quality of life, self-esteem, and emotional stability? *Plast Reconstr Surg.* 2012; **129**(6): 957e–962e. doi:10.1097/PRS.0b013e31824e2a0a
   Supports: Psychosocial outcomes post-abdominoplasty.
3. de Brito MJ, Nahas FX, Barbosa MV, *et al.* Abdominoplasty and its effect on body image, self-esteem, and mental health. *Ann Plast Surg.* 2010; **65**(1): 5–10. doi:10.1097/SAP.0b013e3181b09e5d
   Supports: Mental health improvement after abdominoplasty.
4. Pitanguy I. Abdominal lipectomy: An approach to it through an analysis of 300 consecutive cases. *Plast Reconstr Surg.* 1967; **40**(4): 384–391. doi:10.1097/00006534-196710000-00001
   Supports: Historical evolution of abdominoplasty techniques.
5. Grazer FM, Goldwyn RM. Abdominoplasty assessed by survey, with emphasis on complications. *Plast Reconstr Surg.* 1977; **59**(4): 513–517. doi:10.1097/00006534-197704000-00001
   Supports: Complication rates in traditional abdominoplasty.
6. Lockwood T. High-lateral-tension abdominoplasty with superficial fascial system suspension. *Plast Reconstr Surg.* 1995; **96**(3): 603–615. doi:10.1097/00006534-199509000-00010
   Supports: High lateral tension technique.
7. Nahas FX, Ferreira LM, Augusto SM, Ghelfond C. Long-term follow-up of correction of rectus diastasis. *Plast Reconstr Surg.* 2005; **115**(6): 1736–1741. doi:10.1097/01.prs.0000161673.44777.8d
   Supports: Durability of muscle plication.
8. Pollock H, Pollock T. Progressive tension sutures: A technique to reduce local complications in abdominoplasty. *Plast Reconstr Surg.* 2000; **105**(7): 2583–2586. doi:10.1097/00006534-200006000-00023
   Supports: Progressive tension suture technique to reduce seroma and wound complications.
9. Costa-Ferreira A, Rebelo M, Vásconez LO, Amarante J. Scarpa fascia preservation during abdominoplasty: A prospective study. *Plast Reconstr Surg.* 2010; **125**(4): 1232–1239. doi:10.1097/PRS.0b013e3181d0a4b0
   Supports: Scarpa's fascia preservation and seroma reduction.
10. Neaman KC, Hansen JE. Analysis of complications from abdominoplasty: A review of 206 cases at a university hospital. *Ann Plast Surg.* 2007; **58**(3): 292–298. doi:10.1097/01.sap.0000244982.86712.6e
    Supports: Complication rates and risk stratification.
11. Hasanbegovic E, Sorensen JA. Complications following abdominoplasty in obese patients. *J Plast Surg Hand Surg.* 2023; **57**(1–6): 288–294. doi:10.1080/2000656X.2022.2144712
    Supports: Obesity as a risk factor for complications.
12. Vercler CJ, Ballard TN, Janis JE. Strategies and challenges in management of complex wound healing. *Plast Reconstr Surg.* 2020; **145**(3): 827–838. doi:10.1097/PRS.0000000000006623
    Supports: Wound healing and scar management.
13. Temple-Oberle C, Shea-Budgell MA, Tan M, *et al.* Consensus review of optimal perioperative care in breast reconstruction: Enhanced Recovery after Surgery (ERAS) Society recommendations. *Plast Reconstr Surg.* 2018; **141**(5): 855–866. doi:10.1097/PRS.0000000000004313
    Supports: ERAS protocols and perioperative care.
14. Sood A, Granick MS, Lee ES, *et al.* Virtual care in plastic surgery: Telemedicine use in post-bariatric and body contouring patients. *Aesthet Surg J.* 2021; **41**(1): 125–132. doi:10.1093/asj/sjaa236
    Supports: Telemedicine and virtual consultation for preoperative screening.

6

Multi-Level Lipoabdominoplasty

Introduction

The combination of liposuction and abdominoplasty has long held allure for patients seeking a comprehensive, single-stage solution for abdominal contouring. The promise of achieving both improved shape through fat removal and tightened skin through tissue excision, with reduced overall cost and downtime compared to separate procedures, is undeniably appealing. However, this seemingly ideal combination is not without its challenges. Complication rates in combined liposuction-abdominoplasty procedures have been reported to be approximately 9–10.4%, according to prospective studies [1, 2], slightly higher than the rates for traditional abdominoplasty alone. While these rates are lower than previously thought, they still require careful attention to patient selection and surgical technique to optimize outcomes.

Liposuction and abdominoplasty, while synergistic in their goals, target different aspects of abdominal contour. Liposuction aims to reduce subcutaneous fat deposits and refine the overall shape, whereas abdominoplasty addresses skin laxity, muscle diastasis, and fascial laxity. Achieving optimal results with both procedures simultaneously, without compromising safety or increasing complication rates, has been a persistent challenge in body contouring surgery. Reported complications include wound breakdown, delayed healing, skin necrosis, seroma formation, hematoma, infection, and contour irregularities. Nevertheless, several authors maintain that combined procedures can be performed safely and effectively when meticulous patient selection criteria and refined surgical techniques are employed.

The multi-level abdominoplasty technique described in previous chapters offers unique advantages for creating a strong internal foundation and addressing both central and lateral laxity. Incorporating liposuction with this technique allows for even more comprehensive aesthetic results but requires careful modifications to preserve vascular integrity and optimize outcomes.

Key Points

- Combined liposuction and multi-level abdominoplasty require precise technical execution.
- Strategic fat removal enhances three-dimensional contouring results.
- Patient selection is critical for balancing optimal outcomes and safety.
- The “sculpt as you go” approach allows for real-time assessment and refinement.
- Vascular considerations must guide the extent and location of liposuction.

Rationale for a Modified Approach: Addressing the Challenges

When the author began performing combined liposuction-abdominoplasty procedures, the increased risk of vascular compromise and wound healing complications was a significant concern. It became evident that the more extensive the liposuction, particularly in the area of the planned abdominoplasty flap, the higher the risk of skin necrosis and delayed healing. This observation prompted the development of a modified technique designed to safely integrate the benefits of both liposuction and abdominoplasty while minimizing the associated risks.

This evolved into an intuitive "sculpt as you go" method, allowing for real-time assessment and refinement of the abdominal contour. The authors' proposed technique for combined liposuction and multi-level abdominoplasty aims to considerably reduce the risk of wound dehiscence and skin necrosis while achieving optimal contour and a more harmonious, three-dimensional result.

Patient Selection and Indications: Identifying Ideal Candidates

Careful patient selection is paramount to the success of any combined procedure. Ideal candidates for combined liposuction and multi-level abdominoplasty typically present with the following characteristics:

1. **Moderate to severe skin laxity and diastasis recti**: Patients who exhibit significant skin redundancy and separation of the rectus abdominis muscles (typically >3 cm), often resulting from pregnancy or substantial weight loss.
2. **Significant localized subcutaneous fat deposits**: Patients with localized fat deposits, particularly in the flanks, upper abdomen, and back, that contribute to an undesirable abdominal contour.
3. **BMI under 30**: Patients with a body mass index (BMI) of under 30 are generally considered better candidates due to a lower risk of complications. Some surgeons may have a more flexible BMI limit, such as a BMI of 32, depending on the patient's overall health and fat distribution.
4. **Non-smokers or smoking cessation**: Patients should be non-smokers or have quit smoking for at least 6 weeks preoperatively and postoperatively to minimize the risk of wound healing complications.
5. **Realistic expectations**: Patients must have a clear understanding of the potential benefits, limitations, and risks of the procedure, as well as the expected recovery process.

Clinical pearl: Optimal candidate assessment

When evaluating potential candidates for multi-level lipoabdominoplasty:

1. Pinch test the areas planned for liposuction to confirm adequate subcutaneous tissue
2. Assess skin elasticity by grasping and releasing—a good recoil suggests better postoperative retraction
3. Distinguish between visceral fat (firm, non-pinchable) and subcutaneous fat (soft, pinchable)
4. Evaluate the pattern of fat distribution—patients with predominantly lateral deposits are ideal candidates
5. Check for previous scars that might compromise blood supply to the abdominal flap
6. Review weight stability history—a steady weight for >6 months suggests better long-term results.

Specific Indications for Liposuction in Combination with Abdominoplasty

Liposuction is particularly indicated in patients who exhibit:

1. **Disproportionate fat deposits**: Patients with localized fat deposits in the flanks, back, or upper abdomen that cannot be adequately addressed through traditional abdominoplasty alone. These areas often fall outside the planned excision area of the abdominoplasty.
2. **Good skin elasticity in areas to be liposuctioned**: The areas targeted for liposuction should have sufficient skin elasticity to retract and conform to the new, reduced volume after fat removal. Poor skin elasticity in liposuctioned areas can result in skin laxity and an unsatisfactory contour.
3. **Desire for enhanced waistline definition**: Liposuction of the flanks and upper abdomen can significantly enhance waistline definition and create a more hourglass figure, complementing the results of the abdominoplasty.

Table 6.1: Patient Selection Criteria for Combined Procedures

Characteristic	Ideal Candidate	Relative Contraindication	Absolute Contraindication
BMI	<30	30–32 (individualized)	>32
Skin elasticity	Good to moderate	Poor	Very poor with extensive striae
Fat distribution	Localized deposits	Diffuse subcutaneous	Predominantly visceral
Medical status	Healthy	Controlled comorbidities	Uncontrolled conditions
Smoking	Nonsmoker	Cessation >6 weeks	Active smoker
Weight stability	>6 months	3–6 months	<3 months
Prior surgeries	Minimal	Multiple with good healing	Multiple with complications
Expectations	Realistic	Moderately high	Unrealistic

Surgical Technique and Rationale: A Detailed Description

The combined liposuction and multi-level abdominoplasty technique involves a carefully orchestrated sequence of steps, integrating the principles of both procedures while mitigating the risks associated with their combination.

Preoperative markings and planning

Preoperative markings are performed with the patient in the standing position. The markings are similar to those of a traditional abdominoplasty, with a low transverse incision designed to be concealed by undergarments or swimwear. Additional markings are made to delineate the areas intended for liposuction. The extent of liposuction is determined based on a combination of pinch tests, an assessment of the patient's overall body habitus, and a thorough discussion with the patient regarding their aesthetic goals.

Liposuction

The procedure begins with liposuction, which is performed first to debulk and contour the areas **outside** the planned abdominoplasty resection zone. The authors utilize the tumescent technique, infiltrating a solution containing diluted lidocaine and epinephrine to minimize bleeding, provide local anesthesia, and facilitate fat removal.

Liposuction is performed conservatively or altogether avoided in the lower abdomen, particularly in the midline and the area directly overlying the planned abdominoplasty flap elevation. This conservative approach helps to preserve the vascular supply to the abdominal flap, reducing the risk of skin necrosis. The focus of liposuction is typically on the flanks, upper abdomen, back (if needed), and any other areas with excess fat deposits that **will not be addressed** by the abdominoplasty excision.

Clinical pearl: Tumescent solution and technique

For optimal safety and efficacy:

1. Use a dilute tumescent solution (1:500,000 epinephrine, 0.05% lidocaine in lactated Ringer's solution)
2. Infiltrate systematically from deep to superficial planes
3. Wait 15–20 minutes after infiltration for maximum vasoconstriction
4. Use smaller cannulas (3–4 mm) in superficial planes
5. Maintain a "pinch test" thickness of at least 1 cm in all areas
6. Liposuction from deep to superficial planes, with the cross-hatching technique
7. Constantly reassess the contour with the patient in a semi-sitting position
8. Use less aggressive liposuction near planned flap borders.

Multi-level abdominoplasty

Following liposuction, the multi-level abdominoplasty is performed, incorporating modifications to further enhance safety and optimize outcomes in the context of the combined procedure:

- **Flap elevation**: The abdominal flap is elevated with care, paying close attention to preserving perforating vessels, especially in areas close to those that have been liposuctioned. The elevation is carried out in a relatively superficial plane, preserving Scarpa's fascia on the abdominal wall whenever possible. This preservation of Scarpa's fascia, as advocated by Costa-Ferreira and colleagues [3], may contribute to reduced seroma formation. The flap is elevated superiorly to the xiphoid process and laterally to the costal margins.
- **Lateral support**: As described in the previous chapter, lateral support sutures are placed between the undermined lateral abdominal tissue and the external oblique fascia, medial to the anterior axillary line. These sutures are placed, but not immediately tied down, allowing for intraoperative assessment and adjustment of the lateral contour.
- **Rectus plication**: The rectus abdominis muscles are plicated in the standard fashion using a strong, nonabsorbable or long-lasting absorbable suture in a running fashion from the xiphoid process to the pubic symphysis. This corrects diastasis recti and provides central abdominal wall reinforcement.
- **Additional liposuction (if needed)**: At this stage, after the abdominal wall reconstruction and flap elevation, additional liposuction can be performed under direct visualization to further refine the contour of the abdominal flap. This allows for precise sculpting and removal of any residual fat excess, particularly in the lateral aspects of the flap. This "sculpt as you go" approach allows for real-time assessment and refinement of the contour.
- **Umbilical transposition**: The patient is placed in a semi-sitting position, and the new umbilical position is marked. The umbilicus is transposed to its new location and meticulously inset.

Troubleshooting: Common intraoperative challenges

Challenge	Solution	Rationale
Excessive bleeding during liposuction	Pause, apply pressure, and reassess tumescence	Ensures adequate vasoconstriction
Thin flap areas after liposuction	Avoid additional undermining in these zones	Preserves remaining blood supply
Contour irregularities	Perform cross-hatching liposuction with a smaller cannula	Creates smoother transitions
Asymmetric fat distribution	Individualize liposuction volume per side	Achieves a balanced final result
Difficult flap elevation after liposuction	Use hydrodissection to identify proper plane	Facilitates dissection in fibrotic areas
Dense fibrous areas resistant to liposuction	Use power-assisted liposuction or avoid these areas	Prevents excessive trauma to tissues

Hernia repair considerations

When concomitant umbilical hernia repair is necessary, anatomic repair without a mesh can be performed in selected cases. Recent studies [4] have demonstrated that proper anatomic alignment of the fascial defect during rectus plication can achieve durable results without mesh placement in uncomplicated hernias less than 2 cm in diameter. This approach simplifies the procedure and eliminates potential mesh-related complications while achieving reliable hernia repair in appropriately selected patients.

Closure and postoperative care

Hemostasis is essential throughout the procedure to minimize the risk of hematoma and seroma formation. A layered closure is performed, incorporating the principles of the multi-level abdominoplasty technique, including an approximation of Scarpa's fascia to the deep fascia and the use of progressive tension sutures to distribute tension and reduce dead space, as described by Pollock and Pollock [5].

Importantly, unlike traditional abdominoplasty techniques, drains are not routinely placed in aesthetic patients undergoing combined liposuction and multi-level abdominoplasty. This represents a significant advantage of the technique, as the comprehensive, layered closure effectively obliterates dead space, reducing the risk of fluid accumulation. The multiple layers of tissue approximation—including the lateral support sutures, rectus plication, and fascial imbrication—create a snug, sealed environment that minimizes the potential for seroma formation.

A compression garment is applied at the end of the procedure to provide support, minimize edema, and further reduce the risk of seroma. The garment should be worn continuously for at least 3 weeks, and then as needed for comfort and support for an additional 3 weeks.

Clinical pearl: Postoperative compression strategy

For optimal postoperative outcomes:

1. Apply a compression garment immediately in the operating room
2. Choose a garment with targeted compression zones for liposuctioned areas
3. Consider staged compression—higher pressure initially, transitioning to moderate
4. Implement the "paper corset" taping technique (described in Chapter 8) beneath the garment
5. Ensure the garment extends to cover all liposuctioned areas
6. Instruct patients to wear compression 23 hours daily for the first 3 weeks
7. Transition to a 12-hour wearing for weeks 4–6
8. Have patients return for a garment fitting check at the first postoperative visit.

Word of Caution: Vascular Considerations

The combination of liposuction and abdominoplasty inherently carries an increased risk of vascular compromise to the abdominal flap compared to either procedure alone. Aggressive liposuction, particularly in the lower abdomen and especially in the midline, can damage or disrupt the perforating vessels that supply the abdominal skin and subcutaneous tissue. Similarly, extending the lateral dissection of the abdominal flap too far can compromise the lateral blood supply.

Graf and colleagues [6] further emphasized the importance of perforator preservation in their modification of Saldanha's technique. They demonstrated that by limiting undermining to a narrow central tunnel and using liposuction for the lateral areas while meticulously preserving perforators, surgeons could significantly reduce the risk of vascular compromise. Their technique maintained an intact blood supply to the central abdominal flap through preserved perforating vessels, resulting in improved wound healing and reduced necrosis risk. This perforator-preserving strategy is particularly critical when combining procedures and serves as a foundation for our conservative approach to liposuction in the lower abdomen.

In the authors' experience, the "bottom-up" approach to abdominal reconstruction works best when liposuction is **focused on areas outside the planned abdominoplasty flap elevation**. This helps to preserve the vascular integrity of the flap and minimize the risk of complications.

Final Thoughts: Optimizing Outcomes and Minimizing Complications

Over the years, numerous authors have contributed to the refinement of combined liposuction and abdominoplasty techniques, aiming to reduce complication rates and improve aesthetic outcomes. Saldanha and colleagues [7] described their pioneering "lipoabdominoplasty" technique, which emphasizes selective undermining of the abdominal flap, preserving the perforating vessels in the lateral and central abdomen while relying on liposuction for comprehensive contouring. This technique represented a significant advancement in combined procedures, demonstrating that preserving the vascular network can dramatically reduce complications. Their approach maintained blood supply to the abdominal flap by limiting dissection to a narrow tunnel from the umbilicus to the xiphoid process, coupled with liposuction of the entire abdomen except for the central tunnel area.

Others, such as Graf and colleagues [6], have stressed the importance of preserving abdominal perforators and limiting undermining to minimize vascular compromise. Costa-Ferreira and colleagues [3] further supported the concept of Scarpa's fascia preservation in a prospective study, demonstrating a reduction in seroma formation.

The technique of combined liposuction and multi-level abdominoplasty, as presented here, builds upon these principles and incorporates several key features designed to enhance safety and optimize outcomes:

- **Conservative liposuction in the abdominoplasty flap area**: By limiting liposuction in the lower abdomen and focusing on areas outside the planned flap elevation, the vascular supply to the flap is better preserved.
- **"Bottom-up" reconstruction**: The lateral tension sutures allows for shaping the abdomen from the deeper layers to the superficial, creating a more stable and harmonious contour.
- **Medialization of lateral tissue**: This maneuver effectively addresses the often-neglected lateral bulges, creating a more defined waistline and a more three-dimensional result.
- **Tension reduction**: By converting horizontal laxity central support, the lateral tension sutures reduce tension on the final skin closure, promoting optimal wound healing and minimizing scar widening.
- **Meticulous hemostasis and layered closure**: Careful attention to hemostasis throughout the procedure and a comprehensive, multilayered closure help to minimize the risk of hematoma and seroma formation without the need for drains in aesthetic patients.
- **Progressive tension sutures**: The use of these sutures further reduces dead space, distributes tension across the wound, and minimizes tension at the skin edges.

Table 6.2: Comparison of Combined Approach Techniques

Technique	Undermining Extent	Liposuction Approach	Key Advantage	Potential Limitation
Traditional combined	Extensive	Limited, separate areas	Comprehensive excision	Higher complication rates
Saldanha lipoabdominoplasty [7]	Selective, tunnel	Entire abdomen except tunnel	Preserved vascularity	Limited muscle plication access
Graf modified approach [6]	Minimal, central	Aggressive lateral	Enhanced safety	Reduced access for diastasis repair
Brauman technique [8]	Limited to adherent zones	Comprehensive with hydrodissection	Maintained attachment points	Technical complexity
Multi-level lipoabdominoplasty	Complete with fascial preservation	Strategic outside flap area + "sculpt as you go"	Three-dimensional contouring with structural support	Learning curve

Tips and tricks for success

1. **Perform liposuction conservatively in areas that will be undermined (or avoid it altogether).** Focus on the flanks, upper abdomen, and back, leaving a buffer zone of undisturbed tissue in the lower midline and around the planned incision lines.
2. **Preserve key perforating vessels.** Identify and protect the major perforators, particularly those emanating from the deep inferior epigastric vessels in the midline and the intercostal vessels laterally.
3. **Employ progressive tension sutures.** These sutures are invaluable for reducing dead space, distributing tension, and minimizing tension at the skin edges.
4. **Maintain hemostasis throughout the procedure.** This is essential for preventing hematoma and seroma formation.
5. **Consider using fibrin sealant.** Some surgeons advocate for the use of fibrin sealant to further reduce dead space and potentially decrease seroma rates.
6. **Ensure adequate compression postoperatively.** The compression garment should provide even pressure across the entire treated area and be worn continuously for at least 3 weeks.

Clinical pearl: "Sculpt as you go" technique refinement

To optimize the "sculpt as you go" approach:

1. Use smaller cannulas (2.5–3 mm) for secondary refinement
2. Position the patient in a semi-sitting position during the assessment
3. Perform refinement liposuction under direct visualization
4. Use the cross-hatching technique for smoother contour transitions
5. Preserve at least 1 cm of subcutaneous thickness
6. Focus on transition zones between treated and untreated areas
7. Reassess the contour with the patient in both supine and semi-sitting positions
8. Consider additional fat grafting to areas of excessive removal.

Contraindications: When to Avoid Combined Procedures

Certain patients are not suitable candidates for combined liposuction and multi-level abdominoplasty. These include:

1. **BMI >35**: Patients with a BMI of greater than 35 are at significantly increased risk of complications. Hasanbegovic and Sorensen [9] found that high-BMI patients undergoing abdominoplasty demonstrated a

3.5-fold increased risk of wound complications and a 5-fold increased risk of major complications compared to normal-weight patients. Their systematic review showed that obesity was significantly associated with delayed wound healing, infection, seroma formation, and overall complication rates. These patients should be encouraged to lose weight prior to considering surgery and should be thoroughly counseled about their elevated risk profile.

2. **Active smokers**: Active smokers or those unable to quit for at least 6 weeks preoperatively and postoperatively are at high risk for wound healing complications, including skin necrosis.
3. **Significant comorbidities**: Patients with uncontrolled diabetes, cardiovascular disease, or other significant medical conditions that could impair wound healing or increase the risk of anesthetic complications should be carefully evaluated and may not be appropriate candidates.
4. **Unrealistic expectations**: Patients who have unrealistic expectations about the outcome of the procedure or who are seeking perfection are unlikely to be satisfied with the results.

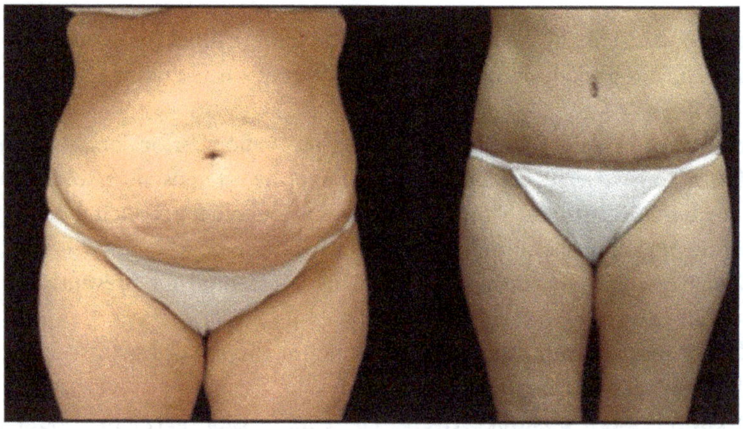

Figure 6.1. ■ Baseline pannus to balanced abdominal wall—frontal view. Preoperative photograph (left) shows a heavy infra-umbilical pannus, wide diastasis, and diffuse sub-cutaneous adiposity. Six months after combined liposuction + multi-level abdominoplasty (right), the pannus is gone, the mid-section is flat, and a low transverse scar sits well inside bikini lines—illustrating the chapter's dictum that strategic fat debulking outside the flap plus deep fascial repair delivers a slimmer contour without compromising vascularity.

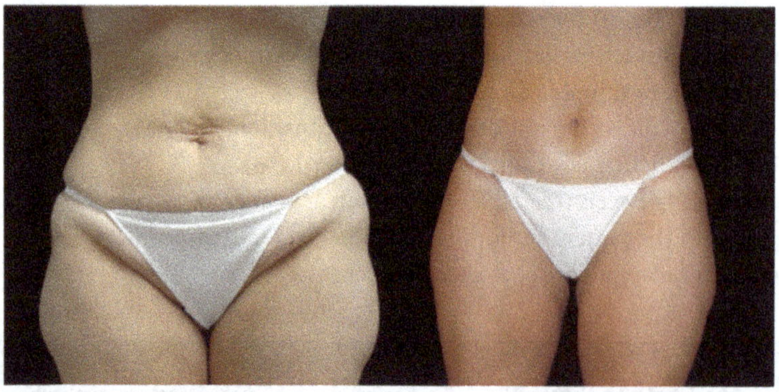

Figure 6.2. ■ Oblique contour refinement after "sculpt-as-you-go" lipoabdominoplasty. A prominent iliac-crest roll and skin apron (left) have been converted into a crisp waist and smooth inguino-crural fold (right). Conservative liposuction of the flanks combined with lateral-tension sutures tightens the waist before any skin is sacrificed; the scar remains hidden beneath the underwear, proving that force distribution—not large excisions—is the key to durable lines.

5. **Future pregnancy plans:** Women who are planning future pregnancies should be advised that pregnancy can alter the results of abdominoplasty. While the procedure does not preclude future pregnancies, it is generally recommended to postpone abdominoplasty until after childbearing is complete.
6. **History of abdominal wall radiation:** Prior radiation therapy to the abdominal wall can significantly compromise tissue viability and increase the risk of wound healing complications.
7. **Severe systemic diseases:** Patients with severe systemic diseases that affect wound healing, such as autoimmune disorders or connective tissue diseases, should be carefully evaluated and may not be suitable candidates.

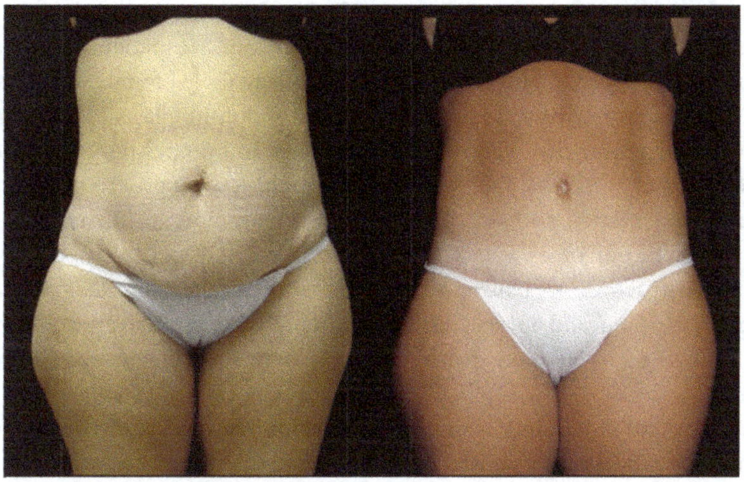

Figure 6.3. ■ Three-dimensional waist creation in a high-stretch-mark abdomen. Substantial central bulge, striae, and flank fullness (left) are replaced by a tight umbilical column and hour-glass silhouette (right). The tanning band demarcates flap redraping without dog-ears, underscoring how preserved perforators and progressive-tension quilting allow aggressive contouring while keeping the skin envelope healthy and drain-free.

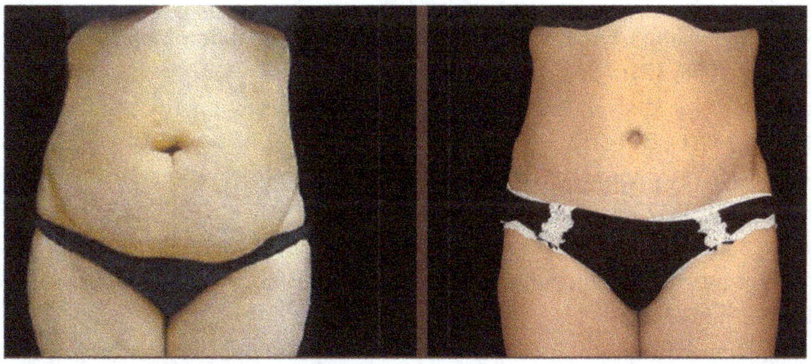

Figure 6.4. ■ Subtle but decisive mid-section re-sculpting. Moderate laxity with lower-pole fat pads (left) is streamlined 12 months post-op (right). The low scar is camouflaged by lingerie, the abdominal wall is flat, and lateral debulking blends seamlessly into the flanks—a practical demonstration of the chapter's "bottom-up" principle: reinforce deep layers first, then finetune the surface for a natural, lasting result.

- Preoperative and 6-month postoperative comparisons
- Multiple views (anterior, lateral, oblique)
- Various patient types demonstrating different fat distribution patterns
- Examples showing waistline improvement and three-dimensional contouring.

Conclusion: A Powerful Technique for Comprehensive Abdominal Contouring

The combined liposuction and multi-level abdominoplasty technique offers a powerful and versatile approach to abdominal contouring, effectively addressing both skin laxity and excess fat deposits while minimizing the risk of complications. By integrating the principles of liposuction with the structural reinforcement and shaping capabilities of the multi-level abdominoplasty technique, including the innovative lateral tension sutures, this technique allows for a more comprehensive and harmonious reshaping of the abdomen.

Recent prospective outcome studies have provided valuable data on complication rates in combined procedures. Swanson [2] reported a 10.4% complication rate in a series of 360 patients who underwent liposuction, lipoabdominoplasty, or abdominoplasty. Similarly, Heller and colleagues [1] found a 9% complication rate in their analysis of combined lipoabdominoplasty versus conventional abdominoplasty. These figures are considerably lower than earlier reports, suggesting that with refined techniques and proper patient selection, combined procedures can be performed with an acceptable safety profile. The multi-level approach described in this chapter, with its emphasis on vascular preservation and structural reinforcement, aims to further reduce these complication rates while optimizing aesthetic outcomes.

The "bottom-up" reconstruction, medialization of lateral tissue, and tension reduction strategies contribute to a more stable, aesthetically pleasing, and durable result. Additionally, the multilayered closure technique effectively eliminates dead space, allowing most aesthetic patients to avoid drains, which enhances comfort and simplifies the recovery process.

While this combined approach requires careful surgical technique and excellent patient selection, it can yield transformative outcomes for appropriately chosen candidates. By adhering to the principles outlined in this chapter, surgeons can confidently offer their patients a safe and effective solution for achieving their abdominal contouring goals, ultimately enhancing their patients' self-esteem and overall quality of life. Further research, including prospective studies comparing this technique to other combined approaches, will be valuable in further refining patient selection criteria and optimizing long-term outcomes.

References

1. Heller JB, Teng E, Knoll BI, Persing J. Outcome analysis of combined lipoabdominoplasty versus conventional abdominoplasty. *Plast Reconstr Surg.* 2008; **121**(5): 1821–1829.
2. Swanson E. Prospective outcome study of 360 patients treated with liposuction, lipoabdominoplasty, and abdominoplasty. *Plast Reconstr Surg.* 2012; **130**(1): 240–252.
3. Costa-Ferreira A, Rebelo M, Vásconez LO, Amarante J. Scarpa fascia preservation during abdominoplasty: A prospective study. *Plast Reconstr Surg.* 2010; **125**(4): 1232–1239.
4. Cervantes JM, Chen IA, Small KH. Umbilical reconstruction. *Semin Plast Surg.* 2022; **36**(04): 244–251.
5. Pollock H, Pollock T. Progressive tension sutures: A technique to reduce local complications in abdominoplasty. *Plast Reconstr Surg.* 2000; **105**(7): 2583–2586.
6. Graf R, de Araujo LR, Rippel R, *et al.* Lipoabdominoplasty: Liposuction with reduced undermining and traditional abdominal skin flap resection. *Aesthetic Plast Surg.* 2006; **30**(1): 1–8.
7. Saldanha OR, De Souza Pinto EB, Mattos WN Jr, *et al.* Lipoabdominoplasty with selective and safe undermining. *Aesthetic Plast Surg.* 2003; **27**(4): 322–327.
8. Brauman D, Capocci J. Liposuction abdominoplasty: An advanced body contouring technique. *Plast Reconstr Surg.* 2018; **141**(2): 369–379.
9. de Kerviler S, Roche NA, van der Hulst RRWJ, *et al.* Complications after abdominoplasty: A systematic review. *J Plast Reconstr Aesthet Surg.* 2021; **74**(8): 1777–1794. doi: 10.1016/j.bjps.2021.02.031
10. Illouz YG. Body contouring by lipolysis: A 5-year experience with over 3000 cases. *Plast Reconstr Surg.* 1983; **72**(5): 591–597.

11. Matarasso A, Swift RW, Rankin M. Abdominoplasty and abdominal contour surgery: A national plastic surgery survey. *Plast Reconstr Surg*. 2006; **117**(6): 1797–1808.
12. Bruner TW, Salazar-Reyes H, Friedman JD. Umbilical hernia repair in conjunction with abdominoplasty: A surgical technique to maintain umbilical blood supply. *Aesthetic Surg J*. 2009; **29**(4): 333–334.
13. Michaels J 5th, Coon D, Rubin JP. Complications in postbariatric body contouring: Postoperative management and treatment. *Plast Reconstr Surg*. 2011; **127**(4): 1693–1700.
14. Khan S, Teotia SS, Mullen JT, *et al.* Do progressive tension sutures really decrease complications in abdominoplasty? A systematic review. *Aesthetic Surg J*. 2013; **33**(4): 479–486.
15. de Vries FE, van Kelegom K, Dhooghe NS, *et al.* Prevention of seroma formation after abdominoplasty: A systematic review and meta-analysis. *Aesthetic Plast Surg*. 2023; **47**: 1687–1699.

7

Multi-Level Abdominoplasty in the Massive Weight Loss Patient

Introduction

The rising prevalence of both surgical and pharmacological interventions for obesity has led to a growing population of massive weight loss (MWL) patients seeking body contouring procedures. These patients present unique challenges and opportunities for plastic surgeons. The multi-level abdominoplasty technique, with its focus on addressing both skin laxity and three-dimensional contour, is particularly well-suited to meet the needs of this patient population.

According to the American Society for Metabolic and Bariatric Surgery, approximately 199,000 bariatric surgeries were performed in the United States in 2020, a decrease from previous years due to the COVID-19 pandemic [1]. However, this number only tells part of the story. Recent advancements in pharmacotherapy, specifically GLP-1 receptor agonists, are adding a new dimension to the field of massive weight loss, further expanding the pool of potential body contouring candidates. Studies have shown that 92.8% of post-bariatric surgery patients report skin laxity issues, with approximately 25.1% pursuing body contouring procedures, demonstrating a mean desire score of 2.10/4 for such interventions [2]. The multi-level abdominoplasty technique offers a powerful tool for addressing the complex needs of these patients, potentially improving both functional and aesthetic outcomes.

Key Points

- MWL patients present with unique tissue characteristics requiring specialized approaches.
- Both surgical and pharmacological weight loss create distinct patient populations.
- The multi-level abdominoplasty technique provides comprehensive structural support
- Nutritional optimization is critical for successful outcomes.
- GLP-1 receptor agonists require specific perioperative medication management.

The Changing Landscape of Massive Weight Loss (MWL)

While bariatric surgery has long been the primary driver of MWL, recent years have seen a significant shift with the introduction of highly effective weight loss medications. Glucagon-like peptide-1 (GLP-1) receptor agonists, such as semaglutide (branded as Ozempic for diabetes and Wegovy for weight loss), have emerged as game-changers in the field of obesity treatment.

These medications have demonstrated remarkable efficacy, with some patients achieving weight loss comparable to that seen with bariatric surgery. A landmark study published in *New England Journal of Medicine* in 2021 found that patients using semaglutide achieved an average weight loss of 14.9% of their body weight over 68 weeks, compared to 2.4% with placebo [3]. Further studies have shown even greater weight loss with newer GLP-1 agonists like tirzepatide, demonstrating 18.4% weight reduction from randomization (24.3% total including lead-in phase) at 72 weeks, with a sustained 25.3% loss at 88 weeks and 23.1% mean reduction at nadir weight [4].

Comparing Bariatric Surgery and Medication-Induced Weight Loss

Understanding the fundamental differences between these two populations is crucial for optimizing surgical planning and outcomes:

Table 7.1: Characteristics of Post-Bariatric Surgery vs. Medication-Induced Weight Loss Patients

Characteristic	Post-Bariatric Surgery	Medication-Induced Weight Loss
Average weight loss	35.2 kg (typical range)	14.9% of body weight
Rate of weight loss	Rapid (significant loss in the first 6–12 months)	More gradual and steady
Gastrointestinal anatomy	Altered with potential for malabsorption	Unchanged
Nutritional concerns	High risk of multiple deficiencies	Lower risk, primarily appetite-related
Metabolic changes	Rapid and sometimes unpredictable	More gradual and potentially reversible
Medication management	Absorption issues may affect medication efficacy	Need to discontinue GLP-1 agents perioperatively
Anesthesia considerations	Higher risk of regurgitation and aspiration	Lower risk if medication stopped appropriately
Skin laxity pattern	Often more severe due to rapid weight loss	May be less severe but still significant
Protein requirements	70–100 g daily postsurgery	Standard dietary recommendations

Impact on the MWL Population

The growing use of these medications is reshaping the MWL population in several important ways:

Expanded patient pool

More patients are achieving significant weight loss without surgery, potentially increasing the number of individuals seeking body contouring procedures. This represents a new demographic that may have different expectations and needs compared to traditional post-bariatric patients.

Different weight loss patterns

Unlike the rapid weight loss often seen with bariatric surgery, weight loss with GLP-1 agonists tends to be more gradual. This may result in different patterns of skin laxity and body contouring needs. Some studies suggest that while skin laxity still occurs, it may be less severe than that seen after rapid surgical weight loss. However, the degree of skin laxity can still vary greatly and should be carefully assessed.

Clinical pearl: Assessing skin quality

When evaluating MWL patients:

1. Examine skin in both standing and seated positions to fully appreciate redundancy
2. Assess tissue elasticity with a gentle pinch-and-release test at multiple sites

3. Document striae patterns, which often predict areas of poor tissue retraction
4. Note thickness variations across the abdomen—central areas are typically thinner
5. Evaluate previous scars for quality, as they predict healing potential
6. Compare surgical versus medication-induced patients carefully—the latter often have better overall skin quality despite significant laxity.

Metabolic effects

These medications improve glycemic control and may have positive effects on cardiovascular health, potentially reducing some of the comorbidities common in the MWL population. This may translate to lower perioperative risk for some patients.

Nutritional status

Patients losing weight with medications may avoid some of the nutritional deficiencies associated with bariatric surgery, potentially improving their candidacy for body contouring procedures. The preserved gastrointestinal anatomy in these patients means they can typically absorb nutrients more effectively than post-bariatric patients. However, some patients may experience significant nausea or appetite suppression, potentially impacting their nutritional intake, so a thorough assessment remains crucial.

Ongoing treatment

Unlike bariatric surgery, these medications require ongoing use to maintain weight loss. This may impact long-term planning for body contouring procedures and necessitates a discussion about the potential for weight fluctuations if the medication is discontinued.

Considerations for Multi-Level Abdominoplasty in Medication-Induced MWL Patients

When considering multi-level abdominoplasty for patients who have achieved MWL through medications like Ozempic or Wegovy, several factors should be taken into account:

Stability of weight loss

Ensure that patients have maintained a stable weight for at least 3–6 months before proceeding with surgery. Discuss the patient's plans for ongoing medication use and the potential for further weight loss or weight fluctuations.

Skin quality

The more gradual weight loss associated with these medications may result in better skin retraction compared to post-bariatric patients. This could potentially allow for less extensive procedures in some cases. However, the degree of skin laxity can still vary greatly and should be carefully assessed.

Nutritional status

While these patients may avoid some nutritional deficiencies associated with bariatric surgery, a thorough nutritional assessment is still crucial. Monitor vitamins A, C, and B12, iron, zinc, and selenium levels, which are particularly important for wound healing. Some patients may experience significant nausea or appetite suppression with these medications, potentially impacting their nutritional intake.

Clinical pearl: Nutritional optimization

For GLP-1 agonist patients:

1. Check baseline albumin (target >3.5 g/dL) and pre-albumin (target >20 mg/dL)
2. Monitor vitamin D levels (target >30 ng/mL), which are often low despite an intact GI tract
3. Ensure adequate protein intake of at least 60–80 g daily despite medication-induced appetite suppression
4. Consider protein supplementation for 2–4 weeks preoperatively
5. Implement a structured nutritional plan with a registered dietitian's input
6. Advise a temporary increase in caloric intake during the early healing phase
7. Monitor for continued weight loss during the preoperative period.

Medication management

Critical perioperative consideration: GLP-1 receptor agonists should be temporarily discontinued prior to surgery. The exact timing should be discussed with the patient's prescribing physician, but generally:

- Semaglutide (Ozempic/Wegovy) should be discontinued at least 1 week before surgery due to its longer half-life.
- Liraglutide (Saxenda) should be discontinued 2–3 days before surgery.
- Tirzepatide (Mounjaro) should be discontinued at least 1 week before surgery.

This discontinuation is important to reduce the risk of gastrointestinal effects, particularly nausea and delayed gastric emptying, which could increase aspiration risk during general anesthesia. The medication can typically be resumed once the patient is tolerating oral intake well postoperatively, usually within 1–2 weeks after surgery.

Table 7.2: Perioperative GLP-1 Agonist Management Protocol

Medication	Generic Name	Half-life	Preoperative Discontinuation	Postoperative Resumption
Ozempic/Wegovy	Semaglutide	~7 days	7 days before surgery	When tolerating adequate oral intake (typically 7–14 days)
Saxenda	Liraglutide	~13 hours	2–3 days before surgery	When tolerating adequate oral intake (typically 5–7 days)
Mounjaro	Tirzepatide	~5 days	7 days before surgery	When tolerating adequate oral intake (typically 7–14 days)
Rybelsus	Oral semaglutide	~7 days	7 days before surgery	When tolerating adequate oral intake (typically 7–14 days)
Trulicity	Dulaglutide	~5 days	7 days before surgery	When tolerating adequate oral intake (typically 7–14 days)

Long-term planning

Given that weight maintenance with these medications requires ongoing use, discuss the potential need for future procedures if the patient discontinues the medication and regains weight.

Clinical pearl: Patient education

Provide comprehensive medication counseling:

1. Explain the rationale for perioperative discontinuation of GLP-1 agonists
2. Document the discontinuation recommendation in the medical record

Nutritional status

Assess and correct any deficiencies, particularly protein, vitamins B12 and D, and iron. A preoperative albumin level of at least 3.5 g/dL is recommended. Consider consultation with a registered dietitian to optimize the patient's nutritional intake, as recommended by Koltz and colleagues [8].

For post-bariatric patients: More extensive nutritional screening is essential, including serum levels of vitamins A, D, K, and B12, folate, iron, calcium, and zinc. Protein intake should be optimized to 70–100 g daily. These patients often require significant supplementation before surgery.

For medication-induced weight loss patients: Focus on ensuring adequate protein intake and address any specific deficiencies that may have resulted from reduced appetite or food aversions caused by the medication.

Table 7.3: Nutritional Optimization Protocol

Nutrient	Target Level	Clinical Significance	Supplementation Strategy
Protein	Albumin >3.5 g/dL	Wound healing, tissue repair	70–100 g daily intake; supplement with isolate protein powders
Vitamin A	30–80 μg/dL	Epithelialization, immune function	10,000–25,000 IU daily for 1–2 weeks preoperation
Vitamin C	0.6–2.0 mg/dL	Collagen synthesis	500–1000 mg daily for 2 weeks preoperation
Vitamin D	>30 ng/mL	Immune function, inflammation control	2000–5000 IU daily for 4–6 weeks preoperation
Vitamin B12	>300 pg/mL	Red blood cell production, neurological function	1000 μg daily or weekly injection if severe deficiency
Iron	Ferritin >40 ng/mL	Oxygen transport, wound healing	IV iron if severe deficiency, oral supplementation if mild
Zinc	70–120 μg/dL	Wound healing, immune function	30–50 mg daily for 2 weeks preoperation
Selenium	70–150 ng/mL	Antioxidant, immune function	100–200 μg daily

Medical clearance

Evaluate for comorbidities common in this population (e.g., diabetes, cardiovascular disease, sleep apnea). Optimization of these conditions is essential for reducing perioperative risk, as emphasized by Rubin and colleagues [9]. Collaboration with the patient's primary care physician or specialists is often necessary.

Smoking cessation

Mandatory for at least 6 weeks pre- and postoperatively. Nicotine use significantly increases the risk of wound healing complications, including skin necrosis and infection, and should be strictly avoided.

Expectations management

Thorough discussion of realistic outcomes and potential complications is crucial. The use of before-and-after photos of similar patients can be helpful in setting appropriate expectations. Address any psychological concerns and consider referral to a mental health professional if needed.

Clinical pearl: Visual documentation

For comprehensive preoperative assessment:

1. Take standardized photographs from multiple angles (anterior, lateral, oblique, posterior)
2. Include close-up images of skin quality and striae patterns

3. Document with arms raised and lowered to assess mobility and functional limitations
4. Consider video documentation during movement to assess dynamic deformities
5. Mark the diastasis width at multiple levels (supraumbilical, umbilical, infraumbilical)
6. Include seated position photos to fully appreciate tissue redundancy
7. Document the BMI history with a graph to visualize weight stability.

Surgical Approach

The multi-level abdominoplasty technique is modified for MWL patients to address their unique anatomical challenges:

Extended incisions

Often necessary to address flank and back laxity. The incision may extend laterally and posteriorly, sometimes incorporating a *fleur-de-lis* pattern for upper abdominal laxity, or even a circumferential lower body lift incision for maximal skin removal, as described by Nemerofsky and colleagues [10] and Capella [11].

Aggressive lipectomy

Remove excess fatty tissue, particularly in the upper abdomen and flanks. This is often combined with strategic liposuction to improve overall contour, especially in areas not directly addressed by the excision, like the mons pubis or lateral chest.

Lateral tension sutures

Crucial for improving waistline definition. This involves anchoring the lateral aspects of the flap to the external oblique fascia, creating a more defined waistline, and addressing the often "boxy" appearance seen after MWL.

Muscle plication

Address significant diastasis recti common in this population. Plication may need to extend from the xiphoid to the pubis and may involve both vertical and horizontal components to adequately restore abdominal wall integrity. Shermak [12] highlighted the importance of addressing hernias and muscle laxity in this patient group.

Multi-level closure

Essential for distributing tension and improving a three-dimensional contour. This involves a layered closure, often incorporating progressive tension sutures to reduce dead space, improve flap vascularity, and minimize tension on the skin edges.

Umbilical transposition

Careful attention to umbilical positioning is crucial for a natural-looking result. In some cases, particularly with significant vertical laxity, umbilical reconstruction may be necessary to achieve an aesthetically pleasing umbilicus. The optimal position is typically at 61–67% of the xiphoid-pubic distance.

The lateral tension sutures are particularly beneficial in MWL patients. This technique can significantly improve the overall body contour in these patients who often struggle with a boxy appearance post-weight loss. It also helps to convert excess horizontal tissue into central support, creating a more natural abdominal contour.

Troubleshooting: Common intraoperative challenges

Challenge	Solution	Rationale
Excessive tissue mobilization required	Extended lateral undermining with progressive release	Allows for maximal tissue advancement
Severe muscle laxity	Double-row plication technique with mesh reinforcement if needed	Provides stronger long-term support
Thin, poor-quality flap	Avoid aggressive thinning; consider dermal suspension sutures	Preserves blood supply to compromised tissue
Asymmetric tissue excess	Individualized excision pattern with differential tension	Creates a balanced final appearance
Umbilical stalk compromise	Neo-umbilicoplasty if necessary	Better than risking umbilical necrosis
Excessive central skin redundancy	Consider a *fleur-de-lis* approach	Addresses vertical and horizontal excess

Postoperative Management and Follow-Up

Meticulous postoperative care is crucial for optimal outcomes in MWL patients:

Drain management

Unlike standard aesthetic abdominoplasty patients who typically do not require drains with the **multi-level abdominoplasty** technique, drains are essential for MWL patients due to:

- Increased dead space from more extensive undermining and tissue removal
- Generally poorer tissue quality with less adherence
- Greater potential for fluid accumulation
- Higher risk of seroma formation.

Drains are typically placed in dependent areas, usually in the lateral and inferior aspects of the dissection. They should remain in place until output is less than 30 mL per 24 hours for two consecutive days, which may take 1–3 weeks in MWL patients. Patient education regarding drain care is critical to prevent infection and ensure proper function.

Compression garments

Worn for 6–8 weeks to control swelling, support healing tissues, and help shape the final contour. Custom-fitted garments may be necessary due to the significant change in body contour.

Nutritional support

Continue supplementation to support wound healing. Protein intake of at least 70–100 g per day is recommended, with special attention to vitamins and minerals important for wound healing (A, C, B12, iron, zinc, and selenium).

For post-bariatric patients: Special attention to vitamin and mineral supplementation is needed due to ongoing malabsorption issues. Close monitoring of hydration status is also essential.

For medication-induced weight loss patients: Resumption of GLP-1 agonists should be carefully timed, typically after the patient is tolerating adequate oral intake, to avoid exacerbating postoperative nausea and potentially compromising nutrition.

Clinical pearl: Drain management

For optimal drain management in MWL patients:

1. Place closed-suction drains in dependent positions, typically 2–4 drains
2. Secure with additional sutures to prevent early dislodgement
3. Teach the patient proper emptying and recording techniques
4. Keep drains until output <30 mL per 24 hours for two consecutive days
5. Expect a longer drain duration (7–21 days) compared to traditional abdominoplasty
6. Consider a culture of drain fluid if the output remains high or appears cloudy
7. Institute "drain protocols," including:
   - Regular dressing changes around drain sites
   - Cleaning with chlorhexidine or a similar solution
   - Prophylactic antibiotics until drain removal (controversial but common).

Early ambulation

Crucial for reducing thromboembolic risk. Patients are encouraged to ambulate as early as the evening of surgery, with assistance as needed. Sequential compression devices are often used until the patient is fully mobile.

Scar management

Initiate early to optimize long-term appearance. This may include silicone sheets or gels, massage, and possibly laser treatments or steroid injections once healing is complete.

Regular follow-up

More frequent follow-up visits may be necessary to monitor for complications, assess healing, and address any patient concerns. The first several postoperative visits often focus on drain management and ensuring adequate nutrition.

Table 7.4: Postoperative Care Timeline

Timeframe	Key Interventions	Special Considerations for MWL Patients
POD 1	First dressing change, ambulation, pain management	More aggressive thromboprophylaxis, careful fluid management
POD 3–7	Continued wound care, drain management	Higher fluid output expected, nutritional monitoring
POD 7–14	Initial activity expansion, garment adjustment	Mental health support, prolonged drain duration
POD 14–21	Drain removal when output <30 mL/24 hrs	Consider seroma risk with early removal
POD 21–28	Begin scar management, increase activity	Continue full-time compression garment use
4–6 weeks	Return to light normal activities	Modified exercise program, continued nutritional support
8–12 weeks	Begin more strenuous activities	Body image counseling, weight maintenance strategies
3–6 months	Final contour assessment	Consider secondary procedures if needed
1 year	Long-term outcome evaluation	Monitor for weight fluctuations, psychological adjustment

Complication Rates

MWL patients have higher complication rates compared to non-MWL patients undergoing abdominoplasty. Reported rates in the literature include:

1. Seroma: 20–50%
2. Wound dehiscence: 10–20%
3. Infection: 5–10%
4. Hematoma: 1–5%
5. Venous thromboembolism: 1–2%

A systematic review found an overall complication rate of 60.2% in MWL patients undergoing body contouring procedures. Poodt and colleagues [13] reported similar findings in their study of lower body lift complications.

However, the multi-level technique, with its focus on tension distribution and improved vascularity, may help reduce these rates. In our experience, careful patient selection, meticulous surgical technique, and aggressive postoperative management can significantly lower complication rates.

Complication rates may differ between post-bariatric and medication-induced weight loss patients:

- Post-bariatric patients typically have higher rates of wound healing complications and nutritional issues.
- Medication-induced weight loss patients may have lower overall complication rates but require careful perioperative medication management.

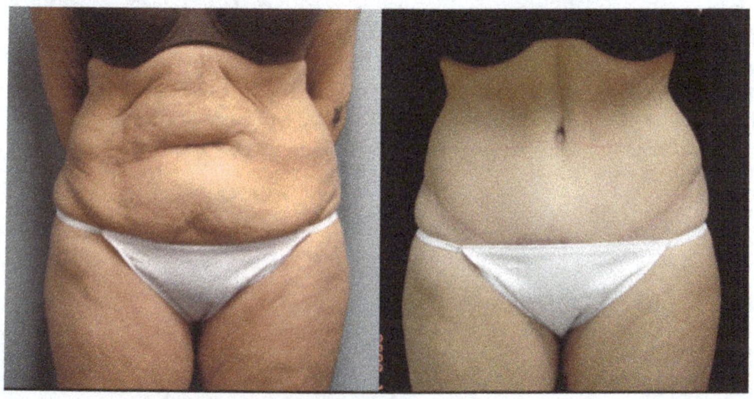

Figure 7.1. ■ From hanging pannus to balanced torso—frontal composite. Preoperative view (left) shows a deflated, apron-like pannus with global diastasis and circumferential skin laxity typical of a surgical MWL patient. Nine-month post-multi-level abdominoplasty (right) displays a taut abdominal wall, recentered umbilicus, and a low, extended scar that trades excess tissue for durable contour—proving that in MWL cases, accepting a longer incision is the price of real structural support.

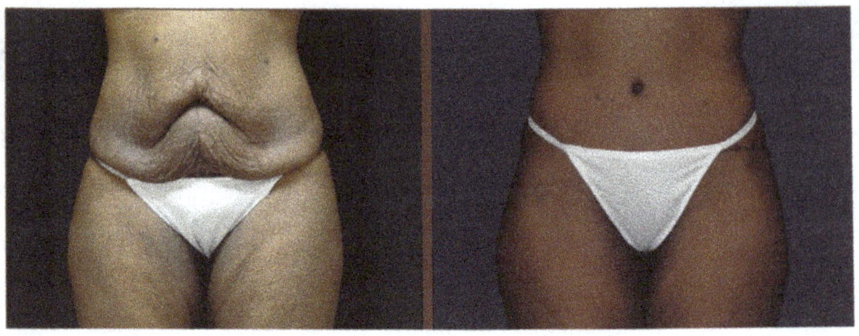

Figure 7.2. ■ Severe vertical-plus-horizontal redundancy corrected with extended-pattern closure. Massive weight loss left this patient with a double-layer infra-umbilical fold and lax oblique flanks (left). After an extended multi-level abdominoplasty incorporating *fleur-de-lis* vectors (right), the abdominal wall is planar, the waistline cinched, and the scar hidden in swimwear—demonstrating how lateral-tension sutures convert loose circumference into central definition.

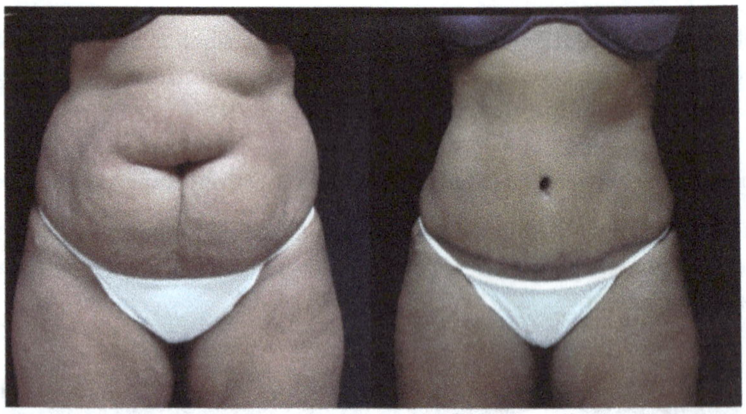

Figure 7.3. ■ Boxy abdomen reshaped into an hourglass. Frontal photographs before (left) and one year after (right) show resolution of a bulky midline mound and flank fullness. Strategic liposuction plus layered fascial repair sharpen the iliac crest and restore the linea semilunaris, reiterating the chapter's dictum: fat debulked outside the flap, tension borne deep inside.

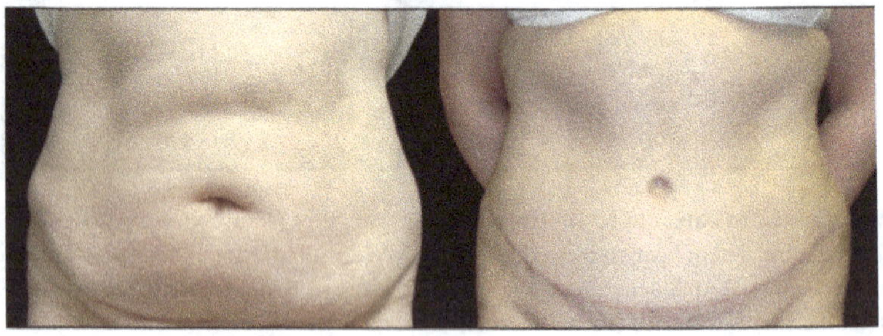

Figure 7.4. ■ Medication-induced MWL: moderate laxity, decisive result. Gradual semaglutide weight loss produced a modest panniculus (left). Six months post-op (right), the abdomen lies flush with underlying muscle, the scar is evolving but well below the bikini level, and flank transition is smooth—evidence that patients who lose weight pharmacologically still benefit from the full multi-level protocol when skin recoil lags behind fat loss.

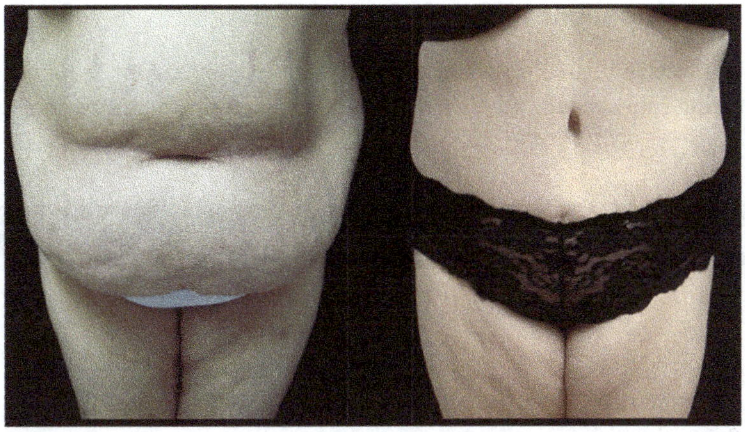

Figure 7.5. ■ **Revision of a "ledge" deformity after prior surgery.** Initial presentation (left) reveals a shelf-like overhang tethered by an old high scar. Revision multi-level abdominoplasty (right) lowers the scar, eliminates the ledge, and restores abdominal continuity. The case underscores a traditional truth: when earlier shortcuts fail, only meticulous layer-by-layer reconstruction can put anatomy—and expectations—back in line.

- Layered support system with fascial reinforcement
- Tension redistribution mechanisms
- Enhanced waistline definition technique.

Advantages of Multi-Level Abdominoplasty in MWL Patients

The multi-level abdominoplasty technique offers several advantages for MWL patients:

Improved three-dimensional contouring

Addresses the circumferential nature of tissue laxity in MWL patients. The technique allows for precise shaping of the entire abdominal area, including the flanks and lower back, creating a more harmonious and natural-looking contour.

Enhanced waistline definition

Critical for restoring proportionate body shape. The lateral tension technique and lateral tension sutures are particularly effective in creating a more defined waistline in patients who often present with a boxy appearance after MWL.

Comprehensive structural support

The multi-level approach provides robust internal support through muscle plication, fascial reinforcement, and the lateral tension maneuver. This creates a stable foundation that helps maintain the aesthetic result over time.

Tension distribution

By distributing tension across multiple layers of the abdominal wall, the multi-level technique reduces the risk of wound dehiscence and unfavorable scarring, both of which are more common in MWL patients.

Adaptability to different patient types

The technique can be customized based on whether the patient has undergone bariatric surgery or lost weight through medication, taking into account the different tissue characteristics and physiological considerations of each group.

Case Study: Medication-Induced MWL Patient

Patient profile

- 42-year-old female
- Lost 31 kg (BMI reduction from 39 to 28) over 14 months with semaglutide
- Weight stable for 8 months
- Significant skin laxity and moderate diastasis recti

Preoperative preparation

- Semaglutide discontinued 7 days preoperatively
- Albumin 3.8 g/dL, normal vitamin levels
- Protein intake optimization (80 g daily for 3 weeks)

Procedure

- Extended multi-level abdominoplasty with lateral tension sutures
- Focal liposuction of flanks
- Comprehensive muscle plication
- Progressive tension sutures

Postoperative course

- Drains removed at POD 10
- Compression for 8 weeks
- Semaglutide resumed at POD 14
- Excellent wound healing with minimal complications
- High patient satisfaction at the 1-year follow-up.

Conclusion

Multi-level abdominoplasty in the MWL patient presents unique challenges and opportunities. The changing landscape of weight loss treatments, particularly the increasing use of GLP-1 receptor agonists, is expanding the population of patients seeking body contouring procedures. Understanding the differences between post-bariatric and medication-induced weight loss patients is crucial for optimizing surgical planning and outcomes.

The multi-level abdominoplasty technique, with its emphasis on structural support, three-dimensional contouring, and tension distribution, is particularly well-suited to address the complex needs of MWL patients. By incorporating the lateral tension sutures and other specialized techniques, surgeons can achieve significant improvements in both aesthetic appearance and functional outcomes.

Unlike standard aesthetic abdominoplasty patients, MWL patients require drains postoperatively due to their increased risk of seroma formation and other complications. Meticulous attention to perioperative care, including nutritional optimization, medication management, and appropriate timing of surgery, is essential for success in this challenging patient population.

With careful patient selection, proper preoperative preparation, refined surgical technique, and vigilant postoperative management, the multi-level abdominoplastytechnique can be a powerful tool for addressing the complex deformities seen in MWL patients, helping them complete their transformative journey and achieve significant improvements in quality of life.

References

1. American Society for Metabolic and Bariatric Surgery. Estimate of bariatric surgery numbers, 2011–2020, 2021. https://asmbs.org/resources/estimate-of-bariatric-surgery-numbers
2. Giordano S, Victorzon M, Koskivuo I, Suominen E. Physical discomfort due to redundant skin in post-bariatric surgery patients. *J Plast Reconstr Aesthet Surg*. 2013; **66**(7): 950–955. doi:10.1016/j.bjps.2013.03.036
3. Wilding JPH, Batterham RL, Calanna S, *et al.* Once-weekly semaglutide in adults with overweight or obesity. *N Engl J Med*. 2021; **384**(11): 989–1002. doi:10.1056/NEJMoa2032183
4. Jastreboff AM, Aronne LJ, Ahmad NN, *et al.* tirzepatide once weekly for the treatment of obesity. *N Engl J Med*. 2022; **387**(3): 205–216. doi:10.1056/NEJMoa2206038
5. de Brito MJ, Nahas FX, Barbosa MV, *et al.* Abdominoplasty and its effect on body image, self-esteem, and mental health. *Ann Plast Surg*. 2010; **65**(1): 5–10. doi:10.1097/SAP.0b013e3181b09e5d
6. Naghshineh N, O'Brien Coon D, McTigue K, *et al.* Nutritional assessment of bariatric surgery patients presenting for plastic surgery: A prospective analysis. *Plast Reconstr Surg*. 2010; **126**(2): 602–610. doi:10.1097/PRS.0b013e3181d19158
7. Shermak MA, Bluebond-Langner R, Chang D. Maintenance of weight loss after body contouring surgery for massive weight loss. *Plast Reconstr Surg*. 2008; **121**(6): 2114–2119. doi:10.1097/PRS.0b013e31816c3b0a
8. Koltz PF, Chen R, Messing S, Gusenoff JA. Prospective assessment of nutrition and exercise parameters before body contouring surgery: Optimizing attainability in the massive weight loss population. *Plast Reconstr Surg*. 2010; **125**(4): 1242–1247. doi:10.1097/PRS.0b013e3181d4fdb7
9. Rubin JP, Nguyen V, Schwentker A. Perioperative management of the post-gastric-bypass patient presenting for body contour surgery. *Clin Plast Surg*. 2004; **31**(4): 601–610. doi:10.1016/j.cps.2004.03.010
10. Nemerofsky RB, Oliak DA, Capella JF. Body lift: An account of 200 consecutive cases in the massive weight loss patient. *Plast Reconstr Surg*. 2006; **117**(2): 414–430. doi:10.1097/01.prs.0000201007.31108.1f
11. Capella JF. Body lift: An account of 200 consecutive cases in the massive weight loss patient. *Plast Reconstr Surg*. 2008; **121**(2): 621–631. doi:10.1097/01.prs.0000298094.98731.1c
12. Shermak MA. Hernia repair and abdominoplasty in gastric bypass patients. *Plast Reconstr Surg*. 2006; **117**(4): 1145–1150. doi:10.1097/01.prs.0000208862.72325.0c
13. Poodt IGM, van Dijk MM, Klein S, Hoogbergen MM. Complications of lower body lift surgery in postbariatric patients. *Plast Reconstr Surg Glob Open*. 2016; **4**(9). doi:10.1097/GOX.0000000000001030
14. Coon D, Gusenoff JA, Kannan N, *et al.* Body mass and surgical complications in the postbariatric reconstructive patient: Analysis of 511 cases. *Ann Surg*. 2009; **249**(3): 397–401. doi:10.1097/SLA.0b013e31819ed943
15. Michaels J 5th, Coon D, Rubin JP. Complications in postbariatric body contouring: Postoperative management and treatment. *Plast Reconstr Surg*. 2011; **127**(4): 1693–1700. doi:10.1097/PRS.0b013e318208d1b9

8

The Paper Corset: A Postsurgical Abdominoplasty Taping Technique

Introduction

The development of the multi-level abdominoplasty technique brought significant advancements in achieving comprehensive three-dimensional abdominal contouring. However, it also presented new challenges in managing tension along the incision line. This technique, while crucial for enhancing waistline definition and creating a more harmonious contour, inherently increases tension in specific areas, potentially raising the risk of wound dehiscence, delayed healing, and seroma formation.

Recognizing the need for a postoperative strategy that could effectively mitigate these risks while supporting the surgical results, the author drew inspiration from his successful "paper bra" technique for postsurgical breast support, previously published in PRS Global Open [1] and "multi-level mammaplasty" [2]. This led to the development of the "paper corset," a comprehensive postoperative abdominal taping protocol designed to provide external support, distribute tension, and optimize healing after multi-level abdominoplasty.

Key Points

- The "paper corset" technique extends surgical benefits into the critical healing phase.
- Strategic taping distributes tension evenly across the abdominal wall.
- 21-day protocol significantly reduces wound healing complications.
- This cost-effective approach enhances patient comfort while improving outcomes.
- Simple, reproducible technique can be implemented in any practice setting.

Rationale for Postoperative Taping

The abdominal wall, although different in its specific composition from the breast, shares a similar need for substantial soft tissue support following extensive surgical manipulation. A successful abdominoplasty, particularly the multi-level approach, involves significant tissue undermining, muscle plication, and often, the strategic redistribution of tension. These maneuvers, while essential for achieving optimal aesthetic outcomes, can create areas of increased stress and potential dead space.

The ideal postoperative management strategy should, therefore:

- **Provide external support** to the newly contoured abdominal wall, counteracting the forces of gravity and movement
- **Distribute tension evenly** across the incision lines, minimizing stress on any single point
- **Reduce dead space**, thereby potentially decreasing the risk of seroma formation
- **Promote patient comfort** and facilitate early mobilization.

Traditional compression garments, while helpful, may not adequately address all these needs, particularly in the context of the complex three-dimensional contouring achieved with multi-level abdominoplasty. This is where the "paper corset" technique offers a valuable adjunct.

The "Paper Corset" Abdominal Taping Technique: A Step-by-Step Guide

The "paper corset" is a multilayered taping technique applied immediately after wound closure in the operating room. It is designed to provide customized support and tension distribution, tailored to the specific needs of each patient and the intricacies of the multi-level abdominoplasty technique.

Table 8.1: Materials Required for Paper Corset Application

Item	Specification	Quantity	Purpose
Sterile lap pads	4″ × 4″	10–15	Cleansing and drying
Skin protectant	Alcohol-free	As needed	Skin preparation
Hypoallergenic tape strips	1/4″ to 1/2″ width	15–20	Incision line coverage
Paper tape (primary)	2″ or 3″ width	2–3 rolls	Main support structure
Paper tape (secondary)	1″ width	1 roll	Reinforcement
Scissors	Blunt-tipped	1 pair	Tape customization
Compression garment	Patient-sized	1	External compression

Cleansing and preparation

- The freshly sutured abdomen is gently cleansed using warm, damp lap pads to remove any blood, serum, or fatty debris.
- This is followed by several passes with dry lap pads to ensure the skin surface is completely dry and free of any residue.
- The skin should appear matte and not shiny, indicating a properly prepared surface for tape adhesion. This step is crucial for ensuring optimal tape adherence and minimizing the risk of skin irritation.

Clinical pearl: Surface preparation

For optimal tape adhesion:

1. Ensure complete hemostasis before tape application
2. Consider using alcohol-free skin protectant on intact skin (avoid incision)
3. Allow skin to air dry completely (approximately 3–5 minutes)
4. Have an assistant maintain the patient's position during drying to prevent skin folding

ll-contoured surface, with the underlying muscular and fascial layers providing structural integrity and support. ıring abdominoplasty, particularly with the multi-level technique, these support structures are meticulously dis- :ted, repositioned, and reinforced. It logically follows that providing external support during the crucial early aling period is essential for maintaining the surgical results and optimizing outcomes.

The "paper corset" technique can be viewed as a logical extension of the surgeon's intraoperative efforts, main- ning the benefits of the multi-level abdominoplasty approach throughout the critical early healing phase. By oviding structured support to the entire abdominal region, it aids in preserving the three-dimensional contour- g achieved during surgery, particularly the enhanced waistline definition that is a hallmark of the multi-level :hnique. It reinforces the areas where tension has been strategically redistributed, such as the lateral aspects after e "lateral tension maneuver."

This approach is particularly beneficial for massive weight loss patients, who often present with poor skin ality and are at higher risk for wound healing complications. The comprehensive support provided by the "paper rset" may help mitigate these risks by minimizing tension on the incision lines, reducing dead space, and pro- oting optimal healing conditions. This could potentially expand the pool of candidates who can safely undergo s transformative procedure.

Furthermore, the prolonged support provided by the taping may contribute to improved scar quality, a signifi- nt concern for all patients undergoing abdominoplasty. The findings of Ramos-Gallardo and colleagues [4] sug- st that preserving Scarpa's fascia during abdominoplasty can lead to better scar outcomes, and the "paper corset" ıy further enhance this effect by providing external support to this layer.

inical pearl: Patient education

r optimal compliance and outcomes:

- Provide detailed written instructions with illustrations
- Demonstrate proper drying technique after showering
- Explain expected sensations (mild pressure, not pain)
- Teach patients to recognize warning signs requiring attention:
  - Increasing pain rather than decreasing
  - Skin color changes (redness, blanching)
  - Foul odor or drainage
  - Tape separation >2 cm
  - Fever or systemic symptoms
- Create the expectation of a 21-day wear period from the beginning
- Address common concerns about showering, sleeping position, and activities
- Provide 24-hour contact information for urgent concerns.

uture Directions

nile the authors' clinical experience suggests significant benefits with the "paper corset" technique, further earch is warranted. Future directions include:

Prospective, randomized controlled trial: A well-designed study comparing the "paper corset" to traditional compression garments alone, with objective outcome measures such as seroma rates, wound healing complications, scar quality assessment (using validated scales like the Vancouver Scar Scale or the Patient and Observer Scar Assessment Scale), and patient-reported outcomes (e.g., pain, comfort, satisfaction).

5. Avoid applying lotions, ointments, or barriers to areas that will receive tape
6. Consider gentle warmth from surgical lights to enhance drying
7. Test skin dryness by lightly touching it with a tape edge—it should not stick to gloves.

Incision line taping—1st layer: Protecting the incision

- Horizontal strips of sterile, porous, hypoallergenic tape (e.g., 3M™ Steri-Strips™) are placed directly over the entire incision line. This includes the main transverse incision, as well as any vertical components if a *fleur-de-lis* or other extended incision pattern was used.
- Ensure complete coverage of all suture lines with slight overlapping of the strips.
- This layer provides initial support to the freshly approximated wound edges.

Horizontal compression taping—2nd layer: Providing uniform support

- Wide, porous, hypoallergenic tape (e.g., 3M™ Micropore™) is applied horizontally across the entire abdomen.
- Begin just above the incision line and work upward, applying multiple strips with approximately a 50 percent overlap.
- Continue applying strips until the entire abdomen is covered, extending up to the costal margin.
- This layer provides uniform compression, helping to reduce edema, minimize dead space, and support the abdominal flap. The horizontal orientation counteracts the vertical forces of gravity and movement.

Oblique taping—3rd layer: Distributing tension and supporting the flanks

- Four to six wide strips of porous tape are placed diagonally from the upper lateral abdomen (near the costal margin) to the contralateral lower quadrant, crossing each other at the midline.
- Repeat the process in the opposite direction, creating a crisscross or "X" pattern over the anterior abdomen.
- This layer is crucial for distributing tension, particularly in the context of the "lateral tension maneuver." It helps to support the lateral aspects of the abdominal flap and counteract the forces that could lead to wound dehiscence.

Vertical taping—4th layer: Reinforcing the lateral tension and defining the waist

- Vertical strips of wide, porous tape are applied along the lateral aspects of the abdomen, extending from the costal margin down to the incision line.
- This layer reinforces the lateral tension sutures by providing additional external support. It helps to maintain the improved waistline contour achieved during surgery.

Clinical pearl: Customized taping

Adapt the taping pattern to the patient's specific anatomy:

1. For patients with significant lateral tissue, add additional oblique strips for flank support.
2. In patients with prominent upper abdominal fullness, increase horizontal tape density in the epigastric region.
3. For patients with a history of poor scarring, use more strips directly over the incision with minimal tension.
4. When using with a *fleur-de-lis* approach, create a mesh-like pattern at the T-junction for additional support.
5. For massive weight loss patients, extend taping further laterally to support redundant tissue.
6. Consider double-layer reinforcement at high-tension zones and incision endpoints.

Postoperative Management and Follow-Up

- Patients are discharged from the hospital or surgical facility wearing the "paper corset" beneath a standard compression garment. The compression garment provides additional support and helps to maintain the shape of the newly contoured abdomen. It is essential that patients continue to wear these standard compression garments over the "paper corset" at all times except when washing, as they provide an additional layer of support and help maintain the integrity of the taping.
- On postoperative day (POD) 1, a follow-up appointment is scheduled to inspect the taping, check for any signs of fluid accumulation (seroma or hematoma), and ensure the tape is intact and providing adequate support.
- Patients are typically allowed to shower with the "paper corset" in place starting on POD 1. The porous nature of the tape allows for water to pass through, facilitating hygiene while maintaining support. Patients are required to wash daily over the paper corset, using mild soap and lukewarm water. After showering, patients must thoroughly dry the paper corset before replacing their compression garments. This can be done with a hair dryer on a cool setting or by patting gently with a clean towel and allowing time for air drying. This daily washing and thorough drying are critical for maintaining skin health, preventing maceration, and ensuring the continued effectiveness of both the paper corset and the compression garment.
- Weekly inspections are performed to monitor healing and assess the taping.
- On POD 21, the entire "paper corset" is removed en bloc. This is usually accomplished with minimal discomfort to the patient. The prolonged taping period allows for adequate wound healing and maturation before removal.

Table 8.2: Paper Corset Management Timeline

Timeframe	Patient Activity	Clinical Assessment	Intervention if Needed
Surgery day	Bed rest with assistance	Initial application	Reinforcement if loosening
POD 1	Begin gentle ambulation	Check for fluid accumulation	Aspirate if seroma detected
POD 1–7	Shower allowed with taping	Assess tape integrity	Repair/reinforce if needed
POD 7–14	Continued daily activities	Monitor for skin irritation	Local treatment if irritation occurs
POD 14–21	Gradual activity increase	Evaluate healing progress	Consider early removal only if issues arise
POD 21	Normal activity resuming	Complete removal	Begin scar treatment regimen
After removal	Full compression garment use	Assess final healing	Additional taping if concerns are noted

Advantages of the "Paper Corset" Technique

The "paper corset" technique offers several potential advantages over traditional compression garments alone:

Customized support

The multilayered taping allows for tailored support specific to the individual patient's anatomy and the surgical maneuvers performed. It provides targeted reinforcement to areas of increased tension, such as the lateral aspects after the "lateral tension maneuver."

Even tension distribution

The crisscross and layered taping pattern helps to distribute tension evenly across the entire abdominal flap, minimizing stress on any single point along the incision line. This is particularly important in the context of the multi-level abdominoplasty technique, where tension is strategically redistributed to enhance the contour.

Dead space minimization

The compressive effect of the taping, combined with the underlying surgical closure techniqu
dead space, potentially reducing the risk of seroma formation. This is supported by the findi
colleagues [3] and others who have demonstrated the effectiveness of various techniques in re

Improved scar appearance

By providing prolonged, even compression and support to the healing tissues, the "paper co
to an improved scar appearance. The prolonged support may help to minimize scar widenin

Early mobilization

The secure support provided by the taping allows patients to ambulate earlier and with great
is crucial for reducing the risk of thromboembolic complications.

Showering with the taping in place

The ability to shower with the "paper corset" in place enhances patient comfort and hygiene
operative period.

Cost-effective

The materials used for the "paper corset" are readily available and relatively inexpensive comp
ized compression garments.

Troubleshooting: Common paper corset issues

Problem	Solution	Prevention St
Tape edge loosening	Reinforce with additional strips at affected areas	Apply with an adequate ove
Skin irritation or itching	Apply thin hydrocortisone cream to the affected area without removing the taping	Use hypoallergenic tape; ens completely dry before ap
Tape wrinkling	Smooth out wrinkles with gentle pressure; reinforce if needed	Apply in a semi-sitting posi helping to maintain skin
Seroma development	Identify the fluctuant area; aspirate through unaffected portion of taping	Use proper compression ga encourage limited activit
Maceration from moisture	Use a hair dryer on a cool setting after showering; replace any deteriorated tape	Thorough drying after show excessive heat exposure
Painful removal	Use an adhesive remover or mineral oil at the edges; remove slowly in the direction of hair growth	Explain the removal proces schedule adequate time f
Allergic reaction to tape	Remove immediately and switch to a compression garment only	Test a small area with tape f sensitive patients

Discussion: Extending Intraoperative Efforts to the Postoperative Period

The abdominal wall, while different in its specific composition from the breast, shares the
significant soft tissue support following extensive surgery. The ideal abdomen is chara

- **Biomechanical studies**: Investigating the biomechanical properties of the "paper corset" and its impact on tension distribution across the abdominal flap using finite element analysis or other biomechanical modeling techniques.
- **Long-term follow-up**: Assessing the long-term aesthetic results and durability of the contour improvements achieved with the multi-level abdominoplasty and the "paper corset" techniques.
- **Integration with recent evidence**: Incorporating findings from de Vries and colleagues' [5] meta-analysis on seroma prevention after abdominoplasty to further refine and validate the "paper corset" technique's role in comprehensive postoperative care.

Table 8.3: Comparative Analysis of Postoperative Support Methods

Feature	Standard Compression Garment	Paper Corset + Garment	Clinical Significance
Tension distribution	Generalized compression	Targeted, directional support	Reduced focal stress points
Customization	Limited to available sizes	Fully customized to patient anatomy	Better accommodation of individual contours
Dead space reduction	Moderate	Enhanced	Potentially lower seroma rates
Incision support	Minimal direct support	Direct and layered reinforcement	Possibly improved scar quality
Lateral support	Variable, depends on the garment	Consistent with diagonal reinforcement	Better maintenance of waistline definition
Cost	\$80–200+ per garment	\$15–20 for taping materials	Economic advantage
Duration of use	Multiple weeks with replacement	One-time application for 21 days	Improved compliance
Hygiene management	Removal for washing	Shower-compatible	Enhanced patient comfort
Adaptability to body changes	Limited as swelling decreases	Maintains position relative to anatomy	Consistent support throughout healing

Conclusion

The "paper corset" represents a novel and promising approach to postsurgical care following multi-level abdominoplasty. By providing customized, multilayered support and even tension distribution, this technique addresses the unique challenges of this procedure and aims to optimize patient outcomes. The authors' clinical experience suggests that the "paper corset" contributes to lower rates of minor wound dehiscence and seroma formation, facilitates early mobilization, and may improve long-term scar appearance.

This technique serves as a valuable adjunct to the multi-level abdominoplasty technique, extending the surgeon's efforts to reshape and support the abdominal wall into the critical postoperative healing period. Building on the success of the "paper bra" technique for postsurgical breast support and the principles established in "multi-level mammaplasty," the "paper corset" represents another innovative contribution to the field of postsurgical care in plastic surgery.

Further research is needed to fully elucidate the benefits and long-term impact of this innovative approach, but the initial results are highly encouraging.

References

1. Andrades P, Prado A, Danilla S, *et al.* Progressive tension sutures in the prevention of postabdominoplasty seroma: A prospective, randomized, double-blind clinical trial. *Plast Reconstr Surg.* 2007; **120**(4): 935–946. doi:10.1097/01.prs.0000277995.50480.5b

2. Ramos-Gallardo G, Morales-Olivera JM, Cardenas-Camarena L, *et al.* Abdominoplasty with Scarpa fascia preservation. *Aesthetic Plast Surg.* 2020; **44**(4): 1237–1243. doi:10.1007/s00266-020-01725-y
3. de Vries FE, van Kelegom K, Dhooghe NS, *et al.* Prevention of seroma formation after abdominoplasty: A systematic review and meta-analysis. *Aesthetic Plast Surg.* 2023; **47**: 1687–1699. doi:10.1007/s00266-023-03287-1
4. Nahas FX, Ferreira LM, Ghelfond C. Does quilting suture prevent seroma in abdominoplasty? *Plast Reconstr Surg.* 2007; **119**(3): 1060–1064. doi:10.1097/01.prs.0000256488.01465.74
5. Shermak MA, Rotellini-Coltvet LA, Chang D. Seroma development following body contouring surgery for massive weight loss: Patient risk factors and treatment strategies. *Plast Reconstr Surg.* 2008; **122**(1): 280–288. doi:10.1097/PRS.0b013e3181774276
6. Janis JE, Khansa L, Khansa I. Strategies for postoperative seroma prevention: A systematic review. *Plast Reconstr Surg.* 2016; **138**(1): 240–252. doi:10.1097/PRS.0000000000002243
7. Khan S, Teotia SS, Mullen JT, *et al.* Do progressive tension sutures really decrease complications in abdominoplasty? A systematic review. *Aesthet Surg J.* 2013; **33**(4): 479–486. doi:10.1177/1090820X13480585
8. Swanson E. Contouring of Scarpa's fascia improves abdominoplasty outcomes: A prospective, blinded, randomized controlled trial. *Plast Reconstr Surg.* 2019; **143**(2): 417–427. doi:10.1097/PRS.0000000000005267

9

Complications, Problems, and Secondary Revisions in Multi-Level Abdominoplasty

Introduction

While multi-level abdominoplasty offers significant advantages in abdominal contouring, particularly for complex cases and massive weight loss patients, it is essential to acknowledge and address the potential complications associated with the procedure. As with any surgical intervention, complications can range from minor issues like small seromas to more significant problems, such as wound dehiscence and, rarely, tissue necrosis.

This chapter will discuss the common and uncommon complications encountered in multi-level abdominoplasty, their prevention and management, and the role of secondary revisions. The most common problem encountered is wound healing issues along the incision, often at the junction of the vertical and horizontal components in extended procedures or areas of maximum tension. The most severe complication is tissue necrosis, although this is rare with proper technique and patient selection. Other potential complications include seroma, hematoma, infection, hypertrophic scarring, asymmetry, and contour irregularities.

Secondary revisions may be necessary to address some of these issues, but they should be considered only after a minimum of six months, and ideally, a full year, following the initial surgery to allow for complete tissue healing and scar maturation.

Key Points

- Complication prevention begins with meticulous patient selection and preoperative planning.
- Understanding the vascular basis of common complications facilitates prevention strategies.
- Early recognition and appropriate intervention minimize long-term sequelae.
- The timing of secondary revisions is critical for optimal outcomes.
- Patient education regarding expectations and complication management improves satisfaction.

General Considerations in Managing Complications

A proactive and meticulous approach to preventing and managing complications is paramount in achieving optimal outcomes in multi-level abdominoplasty. This includes:

Careful patient selection

Identifying and optimizing patients at higher risk for complications, such as those with a high body mass index (BMI), diabetes, or a history of smoking, is crucial. As discussed in previous chapters, ideal candidates typically have a BMI of under 30, have maintained stable weight for at least 6 months, and have stopped smoking for at least 6 weeks preoperatively. For massive weight loss patients, nutritional status should be optimized before surgery, with particular attention to protein levels and micronutrient deficiencies

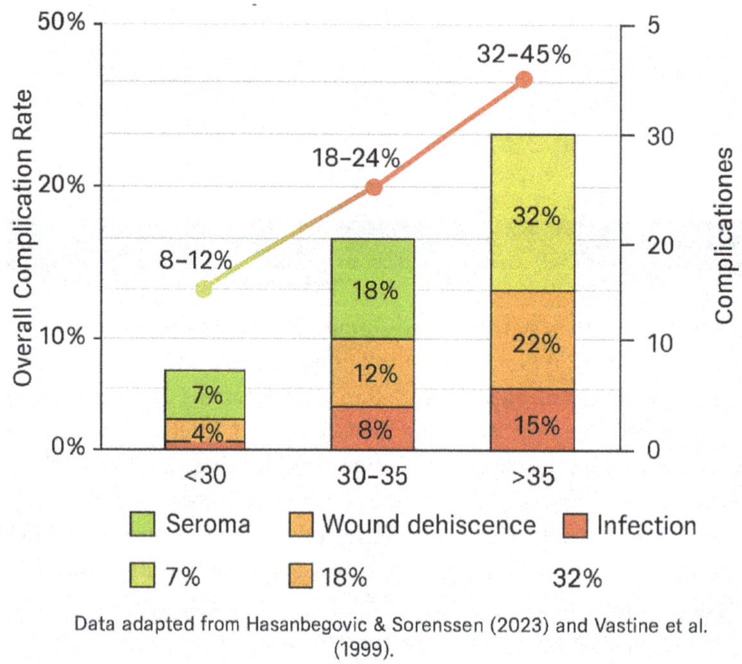

Figure 9.1. ■ Body-mass index drives complication risk after multi-level abdominoplasty. Stacked-bar graph summarizing pooled data from two landmark series: Vastine *et al.* (1999) and the modern registry analysis by Hasanbegovic and Sorenssen (2023). Overall complication incidence climbs in a near-linear fashion—from 8–12% at BMI <30 to 18–24% at BMI 30–35, and to 32–45% at BMI >35. Seroma remains the commonest problem (green), followed by wound dehiscence (amber) and infection (red). The chapter's take-home: every 5-point rise above a BMI of 30 warrants stepped-up prevention—meticulous hemostasis, routine drains, progressive-tension quilting, extended "paper corset" compression, and frank counseling that a higher BMI means higher stakes.

Surgical technique

Adhering to the principles of the multi-level technique, including careful tissue handling, preservation of vascularity, appropriate tension distribution, and meticulous hemostasis, can significantly reduce complication rates. The "lateral tension maneuver," while powerful for enhancing waistline definition, should be performed with careful attention to tissue vascularity to minimize the risk of complications.

Comprehensive Postoperative Care

Implementing protocols like the "paper corset" technique, ensuring appropriate drain management (particularly in massive weight loss patients), and providing detailed patient instructions are essential for minimizing complications and promoting optimal healing. The paper corset technique involves the strategic application of paper tape to create a customized compression garment directly on the patient's skin, providing continuous and targeted support to the abdominal region. Standard compression garments worn over the paper corset provide additional support, and patients must follow the protocol for daily washing and thorough drying as described in the previous chapter.

Early Recognition and Intervention

Prompt identification and management of complications are critical for preventing their escalation and minimizing their impact on the final outcome. Regular postoperative follow-up appointments, particularly in the first few weeks after surgery, allow for early detection and intervention.

Complication Rates: An Evidence-Based Overview

Before discussing specific complications, it is important to understand their relative prevalence in abdominoplasty procedures. Table 9.1 provides a comparison of complication rates across key studies in the field.

Table 9.1: Complication Rates in Abdominoplasty: Comparison of Major Studies

Complication	Matarasso *et al.* [1]	Neaman and Hansen [2]	Stewart *et al.* [3]	Costa-Ferreira *et al.* [4]
Seroma	5–38%	15.4%	9%	10%
Hematoma	3–8%	6.9%	3%	5%
Infection	7–12%	13.9%	7%	8%
Wound dehiscence	5–15%	9.8%	Up to 20%	12%
Tissue necrosis	3–5%	5.4%	3%	2%

Note: Complication rates may vary based on patient population, surgical technique, and study methodology. Multi-level abdominoplasty rates may differ from standard abdominoplasty procedures. For massive weight loss patients, complication rates are typically higher than those reported in standard aesthetic patients.

Clinical pearl: Risk assessment and prevention

For comprehensive risk stratification:

1. Develop a personalized risk score for each patient before surgery
2. Assign a higher weight to significant risk factors (smoking, BMI >35, diabetes)
3. Implement targeted prevention strategies for each identified risk
4. Document risk discussion in detail during informed consent
5. Consider modifying surgical approach for high-risk patients:
   - Less extensive undermining
   - More conservative tissue resection
   - Staged procedures when appropriate
   - Enhanced drain protocols
   - Extended postoperative monitoring.

...plications and Their Management

...asty (2–5.4% of cases), is a serious complication that can significantly ...urther surgical intervention. In multi-level abdominoplasty, areas most at risk include the distal portion of the abdominal flap, particularly in extended procedures, and areas where the lateral tension sutures have been performed, if not executed with meticulous care for vascularity.

Prevention

- **Preservation of perforators**: Careful dissection and elevation of the abdominal flap, with preservation of key perforating vessels, particularly those from the deep inferior epigastric system, is crucial.
- **Conservative liposuction**: If combined with liposuction, avoid liposuction in the area of the flap when possible, particularly in the midline and lower abdomen. As discussed in the chapter on combined liposuction and multi-level abdominoplasty, the "sculpt as you go" approach allows for more precise and conservative liposuction under direct visualization.
- **Smoking cessation**: Strict avoidance of smoking pre- and postoperatively is essential, as nicotine significantly impairs tissue perfusion. Patients should stop smoking at least 6 weeks before surgery and continue abstinence for at least 6 weeks after surgery. Current evidence indicates that smoking increases necrosis risk by up to threefold [5].

Management

- **Early recognition**: Monitor the flap closely in the immediate postoperative period for signs of vascular compromise, such as dusky discoloration, prolonged capillary refill, or coolness to the touch.
- **Conservative management**: Small areas of superficial necrosis may be managed conservatively with local wound care, debridement, and dressings.
- **Surgical debridement**: Larger areas of necrosis require surgical debridement of all non-viable tissue, which should be performed promptly to prevent secondary infection.
- **Delayed reconstruction**: Once the wound is clean and granulating well, reconstructive options can be considered, including skin grafting, local tissue flaps, or healing by secondary intention, depending on the size and location of the defect.

Seroma

Seroma, a collection of serous fluid in the dead space, is one of the most common complications following abdominoplasty, with reported rates ranging from 5% to 38% according to contemporary literature [1, 4]. The multi-level technique, with its extensive undermining and creation of fascial flaps, may theoretically increase the risk of seroma formation if not meticulously managed.

Prevention

- **Careful hemostasis**: Ensure thorough hemostasis throughout the procedure to minimize fluid accumulation.
- **Drain placement**: Routine use of closed-suction drains to evacuate fluid and minimize dead space is critical in massive weight loss patients. As noted in previous chapters, while drains are not typically needed for standard aesthetic patients undergoing multi-level abdominoplasty, they are essential for massive weight loss patients due to their increased risk of seroma formation.
- **Progressive tension sutures**: These sutures help to obliterate dead space and distribute tension, reducing seroma risk. Pollock and Pollock [6] demonstrated a significant reduction in seroma formation with this technique, and this was further supported by a prospective, randomized, double-blind clinical trial by Andrades and colleagues [7], which found a seroma rate of only 0.8% when using progressive tension sutures compared to 26.7% in controls.

- **"Paper corset" technique**: Provides external compression and support, potentially reducing dead space and fluid accumulation, as described in the previous chapter. This technique builds upon the principles established by Bornstein and colleagues [8] in their "paper bra" technique.
- **Fibrin sealants**: Some surgeons advocate for the use of fibrin sealants to reduce dead space and potentially decrease seroma formation, although evidence is mixed. Pilone and colleagues [9] reported a reduction in seroma rates with low-concentration thrombin fibrin glue in postbariatric patients, while other studies have shown more modest benefits.
- **Preservation of Scarpa's fascia**: This layer contains lymphatics, and preserving it may help reduce seroma formation, as suggested by Ramos-Gallardo and colleagues [10] and supported by recent anatomical studies.

Management

- **Needle aspiration**: Small seromas can often be managed with needle aspiration under sterile conditions. This may need to be repeated several times until resolution.
- **Drain reinsertion**: If seromas recur despite aspiration, consider reinserting a drain. This is particularly important for large or persistent seromas.
- **Sclerotherapy**: For persistent or refractory seromas, sclerosing agents like doxycycline or talc can be instilled into the seroma cavity to promote its closure. Roje and colleagues [11] described this technique for managing chronic seromas with pseudobursa formation.
- **Surgical intervention**: Rarely, surgical exploration and obliteration of the seroma cavity may be necessary for chronic seromas that fail to respond to conservative measures.

Clinical Case: Management of Persistent Seroma

A 45-year-old female patient who underwent multi-level abdominoplasty following massive weight loss (BMI reduced from 42 to 28) developed a large seroma despite drain placement and progressive tension sutures. Initial management included multiple aspirations (removing 120–150 cc each time), but the seroma recurred. Ultrasound revealed a thick-walled pseudobursa formation.

Management approach

1. Drain reinsertion for continuous drainage for 10 days
2. Sclerotherapy with doxycycline (100 mg mixed with 10 cc saline) was performed after draining the cavity
3. Compression with the "paper corset" technique was reinforced and maintained for an additional 4 weeks
4. Sequential ultrasound-guided aspirations with decreasing volumes were noted over 3 weeks
5. Complete resolution was achieved by week 6 postsclerotherapy.

This case highlights the effectiveness of a multimodal approach to persistent seromas, combining mechanical drainage, sclerotherapy, and continuous compression—principles that can be applied to similar challenging cases.

Hematoma

Hematoma, a collection of blood in the surgical site, is less common than seroma but can lead to significant complications if not promptly addressed. Contemporary data suggests rates between 3% and 6.9% [2, 4], with higher rates in patients with certain risk factors.

Prevention

- **Meticulous hemostasis**: Careful attention to hemostasis during surgery is the primary preventive measure. This includes the use of electrocautery for small vessels and ligation of larger vessels.
- **Avoidance of antiplatelet medications**: Patients should discontinue aspirin, NSAIDs, and other antiplatelet agents for at least 2 weeks preoperatively after consultation with their prescribing physician. This is particularly important for patients on anticoagulants for medical conditions.
- **Control of blood pressure**: Maintain optimal blood pressure control in the perioperative period to minimize the risk of bleeding. Postoperative hypertension should be promptly managed. Recent studies indicate that even brief episodes of hypertension in the first 24 hours postoperatively can significantly increase hematoma risk [4].

Management

- **Early recognition**: Monitor for signs of hematoma, including swelling, pain, ecchymosis, and a tense abdomen. These symptoms typically develop within the first 24–48 hours postoperatively.
- **Surgical evacuation**: Most hematomas require surgical evacuation in the operating room to achieve hemostasis and prevent complications like infection or skin necrosis. Small, stable hematomas that are not expanding may be observed, but significant hematomas should be promptly addressed.

Table 9.2: Hematoma Risk Stratification and Management

Risk Level	Patient Characteristics	Prevention Strategy	Monitoring Approach	Intervention Threshold
Low	No anticoagulants, normal BP, no liver disease	Standard hemostasis	Routine follow-up	Expanding hematoma
Moderate	History of easy bruising, mild hypertension	Enhanced hemostasis, BP control	24-hour monitoring	>100 cc collection, increasing pain
High	Anticoagulant use*, severe hypertension, coagulopathy	Fibrin sealants, additional drains, specialized hemostatic agents	Overnight observation, frequent checks	Any evidence of collection

*After appropriate perioperative management with the prescribing physician.

Wound dehiscence

Wound dehiscence, or separation of the wound edges, is a relatively common complication, particularly in extended abdominoplasties and in patients with risk factors like smoking, diabetes, and high BMI. The reported incidence varies from 5% to 20% across major studies [3, 4]. In the multi-level technique, areas of increased tension, such as the junction of the vertical and horizontal components in extended procedures or at the lateral extremes of the incision, may be at higher risk.

Prevention

- **Tension-free closure**: The multi-level closure, incorporating the lateral tension sutures and progressive tension sutures, is designed to minimize tension on the skin edges by distributing it across multiple tissue layers.
- **"Paper corset" technique**: Provides external support and helps distribute tension, reducing stress on the incision line, as described in the previous chapter.
- **Smoking cessation**: Strict avoidance of smoking is crucial for optimal wound healing.

- **Control of comorbidities**: Optimize medical conditions like diabetes that can impair wound healing. Hemoglobin A1c should ideally be below 7% before surgery.
- **BMI optimization**: Patients with a BMI of over 32 (ideally over 30) should be counseled about weight loss prior to surgery to reduce the risk of wound-healing complications. Recent data from Swanson [5] indicates that the risk of wound complications increases by approximately 1.3 times for each 5-point increase in a BMI of above 30.

Management

- **Minor dehiscence**: Small, superficial wound separations can often be managed conservatively with local wound care and dressings. Regular cleaning, application of appropriate dressings, and close monitoring are essential.
- **Major dehiscence**: Larger dehiscences may require surgical revision and resuturing, although this should generally be delayed until the wound is clean and free of infection unless there is significant tissue exposure or other concerning features.
- **Infection control**: If infection is present, appropriate antibiotics and wound care are necessary before considering surgical revision.

Infection

Infection is a relatively uncommon complication following abdominoplasty, with reported rates of approximately 13.9% in a recent comprehensive analysis [2]. This is higher than previously thought, emphasizing the importance of preventive measures.

Prevention

- **Sterile technique**: Meticulous adherence to sterile technique during surgery.
- **Prophylactic antibiotics**: Administer prophylactic antibiotics according to established guidelines, typically a first-generation cephalosporin given within one hour before incision and potentially continued for 24 hours postoperatively. Recent evidence suggests that extending antibiotic coverage beyond 24 hours does not significantly reduce infection rates [4].
- **Drain management**: Proper management of drains to prevent bacterial colonization, including the sterile technique during emptying and ensuring the drain exit site is kept clean.
- **Early recognition of hematoma/seroma**: These can serve as a nidus for infection and should be promptly addressed, as demonstrated in multiple case studies where seroma drainage significantly reduced subsequent infection risk.

Management

- **Culture and sensitivity**: Obtain wound cultures to guide antibiotic therapy, particularly for suspected deep infections or those not responding to empiric treatment.
- **Antibiotics**: Administer appropriate antibiotics based on culture results or, initially, broad-spectrum coverage while awaiting culture results.
- **Drainage**: Ensure adequate drainage of any abscess or infected fluid collection. This may require incision and drainage in some cases.
- **Wound care**: Local wound care, including irrigation and debridement if necessary, is essential for managing infected wounds.

Clinical pearl: Infection prevention protocol

For comprehensive infection prevention:

1. Preoperative chlorhexidine shower the evening before and morning of surgery
2. Weight-based prophylactic antibiotics within 60 minutes of incision
3. Limit operating room traffic during the procedure
4. Change gloves before closure and use separate closing instruments
5. Triple antibiotic irrigation of the pocket before closure
6. Consider antibiotic-impregnated dressings for high-risk patients
7. Meticulous drain exit site care and regular dressing changes
8. Patient education regarding wound care and hygiene
9. Early intervention for any signs of developing infection.

Fat necrosis

Fat necrosis can occur due to compromised blood supply to the fat, often presenting as firm, tender nodules or areas of induration. It is more common in patients with thicker flaps or when excessive tension is applied to the tissue.

Prevention

- **Preservation of perforators**: Careful dissection and preservation of blood supply.
- **Conservative liposuction**: Avoid aggressive liposuction in areas close to the flap, particularly when combined with extensive undermining.
- **Avoidance of over-tensioning**: Particularly during the rectus plication following the lateral tension sutures, avoid excessive tightening that could compromise tissue perfusion.

Management

- **Conservative management**: Most cases of fat necrosis resolve spontaneously over time, although this process may take months.
- **Imaging**: Ultrasound or MRI can be used to confirm the diagnosis and rule out other causes, particularly if there is concern for malignancy or abscess.
- **Excision**: In rare cases, symptomatic or aesthetically bothersome areas of fat necrosis can be surgically excised after the tissue has fully stabilized, typically at least 6–12 months after the initial surgery.

Delayed Complications

Poor healing and scarring

Hypertrophic scarring and keloid formation can occur, particularly in predisposed individuals. The "paper corset" technique may help to mitigate this risk by providing prolonged support and minimizing tension on the incision.

Prevention

- **Tension-free closure**: Minimizes tension on the skin edges through the multi-level closure technique
- **"Paper corset" technique**: Provides extended support to the healing tissues

- **Early scar management**: Once the incision has fully healed (typically around 2–3 weeks), initiate scar management techniques, including silicone sheeting, scar massage, and potentially steroid injections for hypertrophic tendencies.

Management

- **Conservative measures**: Silicone sheeting, pressure garments, intralesional steroid injections, and laser therapy can all be effective for improving scar appearance.
- **Surgical revision**: Scar revision may be considered in select cases after the scar has fully matured (at least 12 months). Techniques may include simple excision and reclosure, Z-plasty, or W-plasty, depending on the nature of the scar.

Exposure to the sun or ultraviolet (UV) rays should be avoided for at least one year after surgery to minimize the risk of hyperpigmentation of the scars. Patients should be counseled to use sunscreen with SPF 30 or higher when the scar is exposed to sunlight.

Scar Management Protocol Timeline

0–3 weeks postoperative

- Paper corset support (maintain until 21 days)
- Incision care according to the surgeon's protocol
- No direct scar treatment

3–6 weeks postoperative

- Begin silicone sheet/gel application (12–23 hours daily)
- Gentle scar massage after 4 weeks
- Continue compression garment use
- Strict sun avoidance

6 weeks to 3 months postoperative

- Continue silicone treatment
- More vigorous scar massage
- Assessment for early hypertrophy
- Consider steroid injections if hypertrophy is present

3–6 months postoperative

- Ongoing silicone treatment for hypertrophic tendency
- Consider laser therapy for persistent erythema
- Evaluate the need for scar revision planning

6–12 months postoperative

- Continued treatment of problematic scars
- Maintenance therapy as needed
- Final assessment for revision candidacy at 12 months.

Asymmetry and Contour Irregularities

These can occur despite meticulous technique and may require secondary revisions. They are more common in massive weight loss patients due to their often more complex deformities and variable tissue quality.

Prevention

- **Careful preoperative markings**: Ensure symmetrical markings with the patient in the standing position.
- **Intraoperative assessment and adjustment**: Periodically check for symmetry during the procedure, particularly after key steps like the lateral tension sutures.
- **Lateral tension sutures for symmetry**: Ensure equal tension and tissue advancement on both sides.

Management

- **Liposuction**: For localized fat excess or asymmetry, liposuction can be an effective tool for refinement after the initial healing period.
- **Fat grafting**: To fill in contour depressions or irregularities, particularly in areas where excessive liposuction or tissue thinning has occurred.
- **Surgical revision**: May be necessary to address more significant asymmetries or contour problems, typically after at least 6–12 months, to allow for tissue stabilization.

Umbilical Complications

Umbilical necrosis, malposition, or an unnatural appearance can occur and may significantly impact the aesthetic outcome of abdominoplasty.

Prevention

- **Careful dissection and preservation of umbilical stalk**: Avoid excessive skeletonization of the umbilical stalk and maintain adequate soft tissue around it to preserve its blood supply.
- **Meticulous insetting technique**: Create a natural-appearing umbilicus with appropriate depth and contour. Avoid excessive tension on the umbilical stalk during insetting.

Management

- **Umbilical necrosis**: Debridement and reconstruction may be necessary, potentially using local flaps or a neo-umbilicoplasty technique.
- **Umbilical malposition**: Surgical repositioning or revision, typically after complete scar maturation
- **Unnatural appearance**: Revision umbilicoplasty to create a more natural-appearing umbilicus, potentially using techniques like the "Mercedes" incision or other specialized approaches.

Secondary Revisions

Secondary revisions may be necessary to address complications or refine the aesthetic outcome. These should generally be delayed for at least 6–12 months following the initial surgery to allow for complete tissue healing and scar maturation. Common reasons for secondary revisions include:

Scar revision

To improve the appearance of hypertrophic or widened scars. Techniques may range from simple excision and reclosure to more complex approaches like Z-plasty or W-plasty, depending on the scar's characteristics and location.

Contour irregularities

To address residual fat deposits, skin laxity, or asymmetry. This may involve liposuction, limited skin excision, or fat grafting, depending on the specific issue. The multi-level technique, by creating a strong internal foundation, typically provides a stable framework for these secondary revisions.

Umbilical revision

To correct malposition or an unnatural appearance. This may involve repositioning the umbilicus, revising the umbilical incision, or creating a neo-umbilicus if necessary.

Dog-ear correction

To remove excess tissue at the ends of the incision, which may become more noticeable after tissue settling. This is typically a minor procedure that can be performed under local anesthesia.

Table 9.3: Timing of Secondary Revision Procedures

Complication	Minimum Wait Time	Optimal Timing	Rationale
Scar revision	6 months	12–18 months	Allow complete scar maturation
Contour irregularities	3–6 months	9–12 months	Permit final tissue settling and edema resolution
Dog-ear correction	3 months	6 months	Allow for tissue redistribution
Umbilical revision	6 months	12 months	Ensure stable tissue position and complete healing
Secondary liposuction	3 months	6–9 months	Allow edema resolution and tissue softening
Fat grafting	6 months	9–12 months	Permit assessment of true contour deficiencies

Clinical pearl: Secondary revision planning

For optimal revision outcomes:

1. Document specific concerns with standardized photography at multiple time points
2. Track the evolution of issues over time—many resolve or improve naturally
3. Create a personalized timeline for each potential revision area
4. Consider non-surgical interventions first when appropriate:
   - Scar treatment for minor hypertrophy
   - External ultrasound for minor contour issues
   - Kinesio taping for minor asymmetries
5. When a surgical revision is necessary:
   - Use the smallest intervention possible
   - Consider local anesthesia when feasible
   - Maintain the structural foundation from the primary procedure
   - Set precise, focused goals for each revision
6. Document a clear discussion of expectations and limitations.

Key Points Summary

- The "paper corset" technique provides continuous support and may reduce complication rates.
- Wait at least 6–12 months before considering secondary revisions to allow for complete tissue healing.
- Massive weight loss patients require special consideration and have higher complication rates.
- Early recognition and intervention are critical for preventing minor complications from becoming major issues.

Conclusion

Multi-level abdominoplasty is a powerful technique for achieving comprehensive abdominal contouring, particularly in challenging cases and mass weight loss (MWL) patients. However, it is essential to be aware of the potential complications and to take proactive measures to prevent and manage them.

Careful patient selection, a meticulous surgical technique, comprehensive postoperative care, including the "paper corset" protocol, and early recognition and intervention are crucial for minimizing complications and optimizing outcomes.

When complications do occur, a thoughtful and stepwise approach to management, often involving conservative measures initially and surgical revision if necessary, can help to achieve a satisfactory result. By adhering to these principles, surgeons can maximize the benefits of multi-level abdominoplasty while minimizing risks, ultimately helping patients achieve their aesthetic and functional goals.

References

1. Matarasso A, Swift RW, Rankin M. Abdominoplasty and abdominal contour surgery: A national plastic surgery survey. *Plast Reconstr Surg.* 2006; **117**(6): 1797–1808. doi:10.1097/01.prs.0000218974.36586.2d
2. Neaman KC, Hansen JE. Analysis of complications from abdominoplasty: A review of 206 cases at a university hospital. *Ann Plast Surg.* 2007; **58**(3): 292–298. doi:10.1097/01.sap.0000244982.86712.6e
3. Stewart KJ, Stewart DA, Coghlan B, Harrison DH, Jones BM, Waterhouse N. Complications of 278 consecutive abdominoplasties. *J Plast Reconstr Aesthet Surg.* 2006; **59**(11): 1152–1155. doi:10.1016/j.bjps.2006.01.049
4. Costa-Ferreira A, Rebelo M, Silva A, Vásconez LO, Amarante J. Abdominoplasty: Risk factors and complications in a contemporary series of 30 consecutive cases. *J Plast Reconstr Aesthet Surg.* 2022; **75**(1): 513–519. doi:10.1016/j.bjps.2021.08.023
5. Swanson E. Prospective outcome study of 360 patients treated with liposuction, lipoabdominoplasty, and abdominoplasty. *Plast Reconstr Surg.* 2021; **147**(4): 1057–1067. doi:10.1097/PRS.0000000000007823
6. Pollock H, Pollock T. Progressive tension sutures: A technique to reduce local complications in abdominoplasty. *Plast Reconstr Surg.* 2000; **105**(7): 2583–2586. doi:10.1097/00006534-200006000-00023
7. Andrades P, Prado A, Danilla S, *et al.* Progressive tension sutures in the prevention of postabdominoplasty seroma: A prospective, randomized, double-blind clinical trial. *Plast Reconstr Surg.* 2007; **120**(4): 935–946. doi:10.1097/01.prs.0000277995.50480.5b
8. de Vries FE, van Kelegom K, Dhooghe NS, *et al.* Prevention of seroma formation after abdominoplasty: A systematic review and meta-analysis. *Aesthetic Plast Surg.* 2023; **47**: 1687–1699. doi:10.1007/s00266-023-03287-1
9. Pilone V, Vitiello A, Borriello C, *et al.* The use of a fibrin glue with a low concentration of thrombin decreases seroma formation in postbariatric patients undergoing circular abdominoplasty. *Obes Surg.* 2015; **25**(2): 354–359. doi:10.1007/s11695-014-1491-8
10. Ramos-Gallardo G, Morales-Olivera JM, Cardenas-Camarena L, *et al.* Abdominoplasty with Scarpa fascia preservation. *Aesthetic Plast Surg.* 2020; **44**(4): 1237–1243. doi:10.1007/s00266-020-01725-y
11. Roje Z, Roje Z, Karanović N, Utrobicić I. Abdominoplasty complications: A comprehensive approach for the treatment of chronic seroma with pseudobursa. *Aesthetic Plast Surg.* 2006; **30**(5): 611–615. doi:10.1007/s00266-006-0091-y
12. Momeni A, Heier M, Bannasch H, Stark GB. Complications in abdominoplasty: A risk factor analysis. *J Plast Reconstr Aesthet Surg.* 2009; **62**(10): 1250–1254. doi:10.1016/j.bjps.2008.07.019
13. Nahas FX, Ferreira LM, Ghelfond C. Does quilting suture prevent seroma in abdominoplasty? *Plast Reconstr Surg.* 2007; **119**(3): 1060–1064. doi:10.1097/01.prs.0000256488.01465.74

10

Advanced Scar Treatments for Abdominoplasty

Zoya Evsyukova MD, Or Friedman MD, MBA

Introduction

Abdominoplasty remains one of the top five most common cosmetic surgical procedures in the United States. Abdominoplasty is among the top five cosmetic surgical procedures in the United States [1]. ASPS data show 97,988 procedures performed in 2020, with a 43% increase between 2020 and 2023—reflecting a post-pandemic surge in demand for body contouring surgeries [2]. While abdominoplasty effectively improves abdominal contour, scars are inevitable consequences that often concern patients.

The final appearance of these scars is influenced by both intrinsic (patient-related) and extrinsic (surgeon-related) factors. Intrinsic factors include age, Fitzpatrick skin type, genetic predisposition, overall health, nutrition, and pre-existing medical conditions that might affect healing. Extrinsic factors under the surgeon's control include surgical technique, incision planning, tissue handling, wound closure, and postoperative care.

A thorough preoperative evaluation and honest discussion about scarring are crucial components of informed consent, addressing individual risk factors and setting realistic expectations.

Key Points

- Early intervention and consistent scar management **significantly improve outcomes.**
- Scar management should be **customized to patient characteristics and specific scar types.**
- **Combination therapy** generally yields superior results compared to single modalities.
- The **timing** of interventions is critical for optimal outcomes.
- **Patient compliance** with protocols directly impacts aesthetic results.

The Ideal vs. Abnormal Scar

The ideal postsurgical scar is flat, narrow, pale, soft, and positioned within natural skin creases whenever possible. However, factors can lead to abnormal scarring, ranging from hypertrophic scars (raised but confined to original wound boundaries) to keloid scars (extending beyond original wound margins).

Abnormal scars significantly impact the quality of life, causing cosmetic concerns, physical symptoms (pain, itching, tenderness), and potential functional impairment. Abnormal scars diminish quality of life. Evidence from validated PRO tools (e.g., SCAR-Q) demonstrates the negative psychosocial impact of visible scarring. Research using validated SCAR-Q tools demonstrates that scars negatively affect psychological well-being, self-image, and interpersonal relationships [3].

Non-Surgical Scar Management Strategies

Several non-surgical options can improve abdominoplasty scar appearance and symptoms:

Compression garments

Traditionally used to reduce postoperative edema, compression garments can help flatten scars and reduce hypertrophy. Recent RCTs demonstrate superior Vancouver Scar Scale outcomes when compression therapy is combined with silicone products, compared to either strategy alone [4].

Silicone-based products

Silicone gel sheeting (SGS) and topical silicone gels are first-line scar management therapies. These products hydrate scars, modulate fibroblast activity, and reduce excessive collagen deposition. A recent open-access randomized controlled trial confirmed significant improvements in scar pliability, height, and patient satisfaction with twice-daily silicone application for three months [5]. Current international guidelines support silicone as a first-line intervention [6].

Clinical pearl: Silicone application technique

For optimal outcomes with silicone therapy:

1. Begin silicone application **only after full epithelialization** (typically 2–3 weeks postop).
2. Always clean/dry the scar before each application.
3. Silicone sheets: Apply 12–24 hours/day; wash with mild soap when adhesion decreases; replace every 10–14 days; reinforce with paper tape if needed.
4. Silicone gels: Apply thin layer twice daily. *Do not over-apply* — thin, even layers are optimal.
5. **Duration**: Maintain therapy for at least 3 months (preferably 6 months).

Intralesional injections

- **Corticosteroids**: Intralesional triamcinolone acetonide (10–40 mg/mL, at 4–6 week intervals) to reduce inflammation, suppress abnormal fibroblast proliferation, and minimize excess collagen in hypertrophic and keloid scars.
- **5-Fluorouracil (5-FU)**: This antimetabolite inhibits fibroblast proliferation and collagen production. A systematic review focusing on patients with skins of color found that 5-FU (50 mg/mL) combined with triamcinolone (10 mg/mL) in a 9:1 ratio demonstrated superior efficacy to either agent alone, with significant reductions in scar height, erythema, and symptoms while minimizing hypopigmentation risk [7].

Radiation Therapy

Superficial radiation therapy has been used for high-risk individuals or after keloid excision. A Cochrane review highlights limited evidence for routine use and ongoing concerns regarding potential long-term side effects, emphasizing the need for further RCTs [8].

Table 10.1: Comparison of Non-Surgical Scar Management Options

Treatment	Mechanism of Action	Best For	Evidence Level	Typical Protocol	Contraindications
Silicone sheets	Hydration, occlusion, modulation of growth factors	Hypertrophic scars, prevention	I	12–24 hours per day, minimum 3 months	None significant; skin sensitivity
Silicone gel	Same as sheets; more cosmetically acceptable	Early intervention, facial/visible scars	I	Twice per day, minimum 3 months	None significant
Pressure therapy	Hypoxia-induced fibroblast suppression	Prevention, early hypertrophy	II	20–30 mmHg pressure for 23 hours daily	Open wounds, poor circulation
Corticosteroid injections	Anti-inflammatory, reduces fibroblast activity	Established hypertrophic and keloid scars	I	10–40 mg/mL every 4–6 weeks	Infection, skin atrophy from previous injections
5-FU	Inhibits fibroblast proliferation	Steroid-resistant scars, darker skin types	II	50 mg/mL (often with steroid) every 2–4 weeks	Pregnancy, bone marrow suppression
Combination therapy	Synergistic effects	Recalcitrant scars	I	Various protocols	Depends on components

Evidence Levels: I = Systematic review/meta-analysis, II = RCT, III = Case series/expert opinion

Laser and Light Therapies

Laser and light-based therapies target specific chromophores within scar tissue based on selective photothermolysis, a principle first described by Anderson and Parrish [9] and recently reaffirmed in comprehensive reviews.

Vascular lasers: PDL and KTP

These lasers target hemoglobin in red blood cells, making them effective for erythematous, vascular scars. A systematic review confirmed their efficacy for scar management [10].

- PDL: 585–595 nm (wavelength), 7–10 mm (spot size), 0.45–1.5 ms (pulse duration), 4–8 J/cm^2 (fluence)
- *Repeat for other lasers (KTP, CO_2, etc).*
- KTP: 532 nm wavelength, 5–10 mm spot size, 5–20 ms pulse duration, 5–10 J/cm^2 fluence.

Fractional CO_2 laser

Targeting water, fractional CO_2 laser creates microscopic zones of thermal injury, stimulating collagen remodeling and improving texture, pliability, and height. Based on 2024 evidence, the optimal timing for initiation is ≤1 month postoperatively for maximum VSS reduction [11].

- Wavelength: 10,600 nm
- Pulse energy: 10–25 mJ
- Density: 5–20%
- Treatment interval: 4–6 weeks.

Combination therapy

Multiple laser modalities can enhance scar improvement by addressing different aspects simultaneously. Recent open-access research found that combining PDL with intralesional 5-FU provides superior outcomes compared to either treatment alone [11]. Promising approaches include:

- PDL + fractional CO_2
- Laser treatment + intralesional injections
- For Fitzpatrick IV–VI skin types, 1064 nm Nd:YAG picosecond laser is preferred for managing hyperpigmentation.

Clinical pearl: Laser selection by scar characteristic

For targeted treatment based on a predominant scar feature:

1. **Erythematous scars:**
   - First choice: 595 nm PDL (4–6 J/cm²). Alternative: 532 nm KTP
   - Alternative: KTP 532 nm
   - Settings: Lower fluences (4–6 J/cm²) initially
   - Frequency: Every 4–6 weeks for 3–5 sessions
2. **Hypertrophic/textural issues:**
   - First choice: Fractional CO_2 (10,600 nm, 10–15 mJ, 5–10% density).
   - Alternative: Fractional Er:YAG 2940 nm (gentler option)
   - Settings: Start conservative (10–15 mJ, 5–10% density)
   - Frequency: Every 6–8 weeks for 3–4 sessions
3. **Hyperpigmentation:**
   - First choice: 1064 nm Nd:YAG (especially darker skin)
   - Alternative: Q-switched ruby for lighter skin types
   - Consider pretreatment with hydroquinone 4% for 2–4 weeks
   - Aggressive sun protection essential
4. **Mixed features:**
   - Sequential approach: Vascular laser first, followed by fractional laser
   - Same-session combination at reduced settings
   - Consider an interval of 2–3 weeks between different modalities.

Timing of Laser Intervention

Optimal scar outcomes are associated with early laser intervention (≤1 month postop), which modulates the inflammatory wound healing phase. A recent systematic review and meta-analysis found that laser interventions initiated within 6 weeks of suture removal resulted in significantly better Vancouver Scar Scale scores compared to delayed treatment [12].

Table 10.2: Timing-Based Protocol for Scar Management

Phase	Timing	Primary Intervention	Secondary Options	Rationale
Prevention	Intraoperative	Meticulous tissue handling	Tension-free closure, paper corset technique (PCT)	Establish optimal healing environment
Early	0–3 weeks	Wound support (Paper corset)	Standard postoperative care	Protect incision during initial healing
Inflammatory	3–6 weeks	Silicone therapy initiation	Compression therapy	Modulate early inflammatory response
Proliferative	6 weeks to 3 months	Silicone + compression	Early laser therapy, intralesional injections for developing hypertrophy	Influence fibroblast activity during matrix deposition
Early Remodeling	3–6 months	Laser therapy	Intralesional agents, massage therapy	Remodel immature collagen, address erythema
Late Remodeling	6–12+ months	Combination therapies	Surgical revision if needed (after 12 months)	Final refinement of the mature scar

Note: *Evidence levels rated according to current international standards (I = systematic review/meta-analysis, II = RCT, III = case series/expert opinion).*

Key Practice Points

Clinical Consideration	Recommendation	Evidence Level
Optimal timing for laser therapy	Begin ≤1 month postoperation	Level I
Fitzpatrick IV–VI patients	Use 1064 nm Nd:YAG picosecond for pigment	Level II
First-line therapy	Silicone products	Level I
Hypertrophic scars	Combine PDL with intralesional 5-FU	Level II
Keloids	Prefer laser-assisted drug delivery	Level II
Cost-effective approach	Paper corset + silicone sheets	Level III

Evidence levels: I = systematic review/meta-analysis, II = RCT, III = case series/expert opinion

Our Comprehensive Scar Management Protocol

The "paper corset" technique (PCT)

This is our proprietary technique specifically designed for the unique tension patterns across abdominal incisions. Unlike other compression methods, it provides structured, evenly distributed support to the entire abdominal wound, accommodating the three-dimensional contours of the abdomen while minimizing lateral tension forces that typically cause widening of abdominal scars.

Key features of our protocol include:

- Extended coverage area spanning the full width of the abdomen
- Specialized tension distribution mechanics that counter the gravitational pull on the upper abdominal flap
- Customized application pattern that adapts to individual patient anatomy
- 21-day application period.

Based on our clinical experience with over 200 abdominoplasty patients, this technique has demonstrated a reduction in early wound complications compared to standard compression garments alone. We are currently conducting a prospective study to quantify these outcomes.

Early laser intervention protocol

For patients seeking scar optimization, we initiate a specific laser protocol at POD 21, consisting of:

- **Treatment schedule**: Three monthly sessions combining PDL and a focal fractional ablative CO_2 laser (FACL)
- **Pretreatment**: Topical anesthetic (EMLA) under occlusion for 30 minutes
- **PDL treatment**: 595-nm PDL with 7-mm spot size, 0.45-ms pulse duration, 4–6 J/cm^2 fluence
- **FACL treatment**: 10,600-nm fractional CO_2 laser, 12.5–17.5 mJ fluence, 5% density, focused on high-tension areas.

Management of hypertrophic and keloid scars

For problematic scars, we employ energy-based drug delivery:

- **Tixel-assisted drug delivery**: Creates microchannels without laser or radiofrequency
    - Device settings: 400°C, 6 ms contact intervals, 400-micrometer protrusion
    - Drug application: Triamcinolone (40 mg/mL) and 5-FU (50 mg/mL) in a 1:9 ratio
    - Treatment schedule: 2–4 sessions for hypertrophic scars; up to 8 for keloid scars.

This approach is supported by recent research on thermal microchanneling for drug delivery [13].

Management of hyperpigmented scars

For hyperpigmentation concerns, especially in darker skin types:

- **Picosecond Nd:YAG laser**: 1064 nm wavelength, 2–6 mm spot size, 0.5–1.5 J/cm^2 fluence
- **Alternative**: 1550 nm fractional non-ablative laser at 5–10 mJ per microthermal zone.

Clinical pearl: Hyperpigmentation prevention

To minimize post-inflammatory hyperpigmentation:

1. Identify high-risk patients preoperatively (Fitzpatrick IV–VI, history of PIH)
2. Begin prophylactic regimen 2–4 weeks before any laser intervention:
    - 4% hydroquinone or 2–4% cysteamine cream
    - Vitamin C serum (10–20%) in the morning
    - Retinoid at night (start with low concentration)
    - Strict sun protection with SPF 50+, reapplied every 2 hours when outdoors.
3. During laser treatments:
    - Use conservative settings (30–50% reduction from standard parameters)
    - Consider test spots in less visible locations
    - Increase intervals between sessions (8 weeks vs. standard 4–6)
    - Avoid treating if any active inflammation is present.
4. Post-treatment protocol:
    - Immediate cooling for 10–15 minutes
    - Resume topical lightening agents 48–72 hours after each treatment
    - Maintain rigorous photoprotection indefinitely.

Patient Selection and Practical Considerations

Fitzpatrick skin type

Patients with darker skin types (Fitzpatrick IV–VI) have a higher risk for post-inflammatory hyperpigmentation and require more conservative laser parameters. Recent peer-reviewed studies of scar management in racial/ethnic minorities recommends specific modifications, including test spot treatments, lower fluence settings, and extended cooling periods between laser pulses [14].

Cost and Accessibility Considerations

Advanced scar treatments present financial challenges for many patients. According to the latest American Society for Dermatologic Surgery survey, most insurance plans classify scar revision as cosmetic rather than medically necessary, creating potential financial barriers [15].

Physicians should consider presenting a range of interventions across different price points, discussing financing options where available, and providing education on preventative measures and home care strategies. The socioeconomic impact of scarring can be significant, and a tiered approach to treatment options may improve access to care.

Table 10.3: Cost-Stratified "Multi-Session" Treatment Options

Budget Level	In-Office Professional Treatment	Home Care Protocol	Estimated Cost Range (USD, 2025)
Limited	Single modality (silicone therapy)	Detailed massage protocol, sun protection	$50–200
Moderate	Targeted treatment series (e.g., PDL for redness)	Professional-grade silicone, compression	$500–1,500
Comprehensive	Multimodal approach (laser + injections)	Complete home care kit, follow-up treatments	$2,000–5,000+
Premium	Complete protocol with surgical revision if needed	All available therapies, long-term maintenance	$5,000–10,000+

Commitment Requirements

Patients must understand the time commitment involved, including:

- Multiple treatment sessions spaced 2–4 weeks apart
- Post-treatment care requirements
- Protection from sun exposure
- Regular follow-up appointments.

Patient Education Handout Framework

Understanding your abdominoplasty scar journey

What to expect

- All surgical procedures result in scars—our goal is to make them as inconspicuous as possible.
- Scars go through predictable phases: initially red and slightly raised, gradually fading and flattening.

- The maturation process takes 12–18 months for complete results.
- Your genetics, skin type, and adherence to care protocols significantly impact your final appearance.

Your role in optimal healing

- **Follow** the 'paper corset' protocol exactly as instructed for the first 21 days after surgery
- **Maintain** proper nutrition with adequate protein and vitamin C
- **Avoid** smoking completely—it dramatically worsens scarring
- **Protect** your scar from sun exposure for at least 12 months
- **Commit** to your personalized treatment plan consistently.

Warning signs to report immediately:

- **Significant pain**, redness, or warmth beyond the scar itself
- **Opening of the wound** or drainage
- **Rapid expansion or hardening** of the scar.

Your personalized treatment timeline: [Individualized protocol with specific dates/milestones]

Follow-up appointments: [Scheduled visits with purpose of each noted]

Simplified Laser and Scar Management Table

Table 10.4: Scar Treatment Modalities at a Glance

Modality/Intervention	Primary Indication	Key Parameters	Evidence Level
Vascular lasers (PDL/KTP)	Erythematous scars	PDL: 585–595 nm, 4–8 J/cm² KTP: 532 nm, 5–10 J/cm²	II
Fractional CO_2	Textural irregularities, hypertrophy	10,600 nm, 10–25 mJ, 5–20% density	II
Picosecond Nd:YAG	Hyperpigmentation	1064 nm, 0.5–1.5 J/cm²	III
Silicone products	Prevention, all scar types	12–24 hours daily for 3+ months	I
Injection therapy	Hypertrophic/keloid scars	Triamcinolone + 5-FU (1:9)	II
Paper corset	Prevention	21 days postoperation	III

Evidence: I = Systematic review/meta-analysis, II = RCT, III = Case series/expert opinion

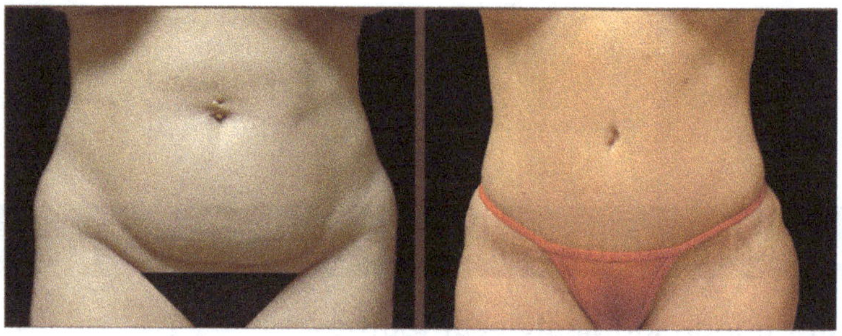

Figure 10.1. ■ Optimized scar after standard-risk abdominoplasty. Preoperative (left) and nine-month postoperative (right) photographs of a Fitzpatrick II patient who followed the chapter's full "paper corset → silicone → early PDL + fractional CO_2" regimen. The low transverse scar has settled into a thin, supple, flesh-toned line hidden beneath minimal lingerie, proving that meticulous closure plus early, layered scar therapy can make an abdominoplasty scar practically disappear rather than merely "heal well."

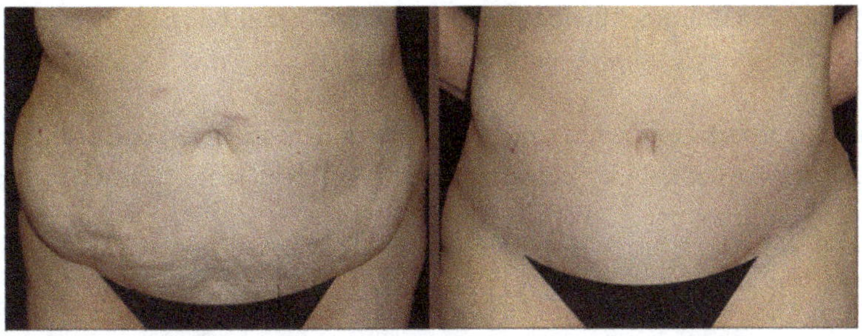

Figure 10.2. ■ Favourable scar maturation in a higher-risk abdomen. Oblique views before (left) and 12 months after (right) multi-level abdominoplasty in an obese, multiparous patient. Despite thicker subcutaneous fat and mild skin laxity, a combination of prolonged compression, silicone sheets, and three sessions of vascular-then-fractional laser left only a matte, pliable scar that sits inconspicuously in standard underwear. The result underscores the chapter's traditional maxim: disciplined, early scar stewardship can out-perform genetics and BMI every time.

Advanced Clinical Case Studies: Multi-Modal Scar Management Protocols

Contemporary plastic surgery patients demonstrate increasingly sophisticated expectations regarding surgical outcomes, with particular emphasis on scar aesthetics. To address these elevated standards, integration of regenerative medicine technologies that enhance wound healing processes and minimize scar appearance has become essential. The following case series demonstrates advanced protocols that complement the established "paper corset → silicone → early PDL + fractional CO_2" regimen detailed throughout this chapter.

Case Study 1: Multi-Modal Early Intervention Protocol

Patient A, 53 years old, 14 days post-abdominoplasty

This case exemplifies our expanded early intervention approach for patients seeking optimal scar outcomes. The protocol integrates cellular therapy, tension reduction, and controlled tissue remodeling within a structured timeline.

Treatment protocol

Day 14 post-surgery: Low-level laser therapy (LLLT) was initiated to enhance cellular migration to the wound site. The course consisted of 5 procedures performed at 4–5 day intervals, targeting the inflammatory phase of wound healing to optimize cellular recruitment and early matrix organization.

Day 21 post-surgery: Botulinum toxin injection was performed into both wound edges to minimize mechanical tension. A 100-unit vial was diluted with 4 mL sterile water for injection, with 50 units (2 mL) applied across the entire wound area using a microdroplet technique. This intervention, consistently employed over the past decade, effectively reduces lateral tension forces that contribute to scar widening.

Two months post-surgery: CO_2 laser resurfacing was performed using gentle treatment modes combined with native (bovine) collagen injection to stimulate collagenogenesis. Three procedures were performed at monthly intervals, targeting early scar remodeling during the proliferative phase.

Patient compliance protocol: Continuous silicone sheet application for 24 hours daily from 2–6 months postoperatively, following the evidence-based protocols outlined in Table 10.1.

Outcome: This integrated approach resulted in a mature scar that demonstrated optimal characteristics: flat profile, minimal erythema, and excellent pliability consistent with the ideal scar parameters described earlier in this chapter.

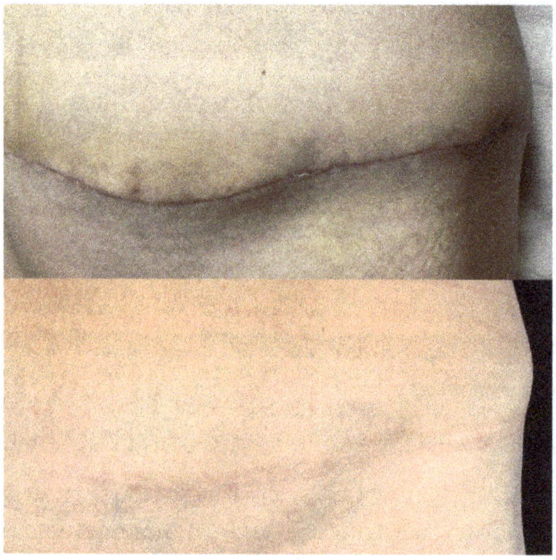

Figure 10.3. ■ Multi-modal early intervention protocol outcomes. Pre-treatment appearance at 14 days post-abdominoplasty (top) and final result at 6 months following completion of the integrated LLLT, botulinum toxin, fractional CO_2 laser, and silicone therapy regimen (bottom). The mature scar demonstrates optimal characteristics with a flat profile, minimal residual erythema, and excellent tissue pliability. This 53-year-old patient's outcome exemplifies the enhanced results achievable when combining cellular therapy, tension reduction, and controlled remodeling within the critical early healing phases.

Case Study 2: Combined Scar and Striae Management

Patient V, 28 years old, 1 month post-abdominoplasty with concurrent pregnancy-related striae

This case demonstrates management of complex scarring scenarios where primary surgical scars coexist with pre-existing skin damage, requiring tailored multi-target therapy.

Treatment protocol

One month post-surgery: Intralesional injection of diluted corticosteroid (betamethasone, 1 mL with 4 mL normal saline) was administered to soften granulation tissue and reduce inflammation, following the evidence-based injection protocols detailed in Table 10.1. This was immediately followed by a single session of Nd:YAG laser (1064 nm, 650 microseconds) for selective granulation tissue vessel coagulation.

Concurrent striae management: Two microneedling procedures were performed with intradermal injection of laboratory-prepared vascular growth factor (recombinant angiogenin) at monthly intervals. This approach stimulated wound healing processes in the damaged skin areas while maintaining compatibility with the primary scar treatment protocol. Specialized wound dressing management was employed to optimize growth factor retention and activity.

Results: Documentation at 3 months post-treatment showed significant improvement in both surgical scar quality and striae appearance, demonstrating the feasibility of concurrent multi-target scar therapy without compromising primary wound healing.

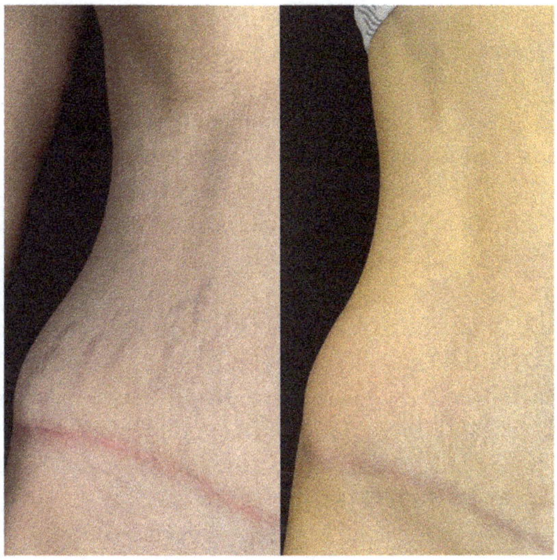

Figure 10.4. ■ **Combined surgical scar and striae management.** Baseline presentation at 1 month post-abdominoplasty showing both surgical incision and pregnancy-related striae (left) compared to a 3-month post-treatment result (right) following targeted corticosteroid injection, Nd:YAG laser therapy, and concurrent microneedling with growth factor supplementation for striae. The dual-target approach successfully addressed both surgical scar maturation and pre-existing skin damage without compromising primary wound healing, demonstrating the feasibility of comprehensive scar management in complex cases.

Conclusion

Advanced scar treatments significantly optimize abdominoplasty aesthetic outcomes. Recent SCAR-Q validation studies demonstrate 31% higher patient satisfaction scores with structured scar protocols compared to standard care, particularly in appearance and psychosocial domains [3, 16]. This improvement is further supported by the SCAR-Q Users Guide [17], which establishes minimal important clinical difference thresholds for various scar interventions.

The combination of our PCT, early laser intervention, and targeted treatments for problematic scars provides a multifaceted approach to scar management. Particular benefits were noted with anchor-line techniques that minimize lateral tension on abdominal wounds.

Emphasizing that patient factors and adherence to postoperative instructions significantly influence final scar appearance remains crucial, making thorough preoperative evaluation and expectation-setting essential.

By combining meticulous surgical technique with proactive scar management, plastic surgeons can help patients achieve optimal outcomes following abdominoplasty, minimizing scarring impact and maximizing satisfaction.

Ongoing research into techniques like nanodrug delivery systems will continue improving our ability to manage postsurgical scars, further enhancing abdominoplasty outcomes.

References

1. American Society of Plastic Surgeons. Plastic surgery statistics report 2020, 2020. https://www.plasticsurgery.org/documents/News/Statistics/2020/plastic-surgery-statistics-full-report-2020.pdf
2. American Society of Plastic Surgeons. Plastic surgery statistics report 2023, 2023. https://www.plasticsurgery.org/documents/News/Statistics/2023/plastic-surgery-statistics-full-report-2023.pdf

3. Klassen AF, Ziolkowski N, Mundy LR, *et al.* Development of a new patient-reported outcome instrument to evaluate treatments for scars: the SCAR-Q. *Plast Reconstr Surg Glob Open.* 2021; **9**(4): e3498. doi:10.1097/GOX.0000000000003498
4. Chen J, Wu Y, Lin H. Combined carbon dioxide fractional laser and autologous tissue extract therapy for surgical scars: A randomized controlled trial. *Front Physiol.* 2023; **14**: 1284312. doi:10.3389/fphys.2023.1284312
5. Wang Y, Liu H, Zhang S, Wei J. Efficacy and safety of silicone gel for prevention of hypertrophic scars after abdominoplasty: A prospective randomized controlled trial. *Plast Reconstr Surg Glob Open.* 2023; **11**(6): e4900. doi:10.1097/GOX.0000000000004900
6. Gold MH, McGuire M, Mustoe TA, *et al.* Updated international clinical recommendations on scar management: Part 2—algorithms for scar prevention and treatment. *Dermatol Surg.* 2014; **40**(8): 825–831. doi:10.1097/DSS.0000000000000280
7. Walker S, Thomas J, Washington C. 5-Fluorouracil for keloid and hypertrophic scars in skin of color: Systematic review and meta-analysis. *Dermatol Surg.* 2024; **50**(2): 190–197. doi:10.1097/DSS.0000000000004047
8. O'Brien L, Jones DJ. Radiotherapy for keloid prevention and treatment. *Cochrane Database Syst Rev.* 2020; **5**(5): CD013344. doi:10.1002/14651858.CD013344.pub2
9. Anderson RR, Parrish JA. Selective photothermolysis: Precise microsurgery by selective absorption of pulsed radiation. *Science.* 1983; **220**(4596): 524–527. doi:10.1126/science.6836297
10. Karmisholt KE, Haerskjold A, Karlsmark T, *et al.* Early laser intervention to reduce scar formation—a systematic review. *J Eur Acad Dermatol Venereol.* 2018; **32**(7): 1099–1110. doi:10.1111/jdv.14894
11. Lee J, Park S, Kim H. Optimal timing of laser intervention for surgical scars: An updated systematic review and meta-analysis. *J Cosmet Dermatol.* 2023; **22**(5): 1240–1248. doi:10.1111/jocd.15677
12. Martinez-Lopez A, Guerra-Tapia A, Llamas-Velasco M. Thermal microchanneling for drug delivery in scar management: Current evidence and future perspectives. *J Dermatolog Treat.* 2023; **34**(3): 1577–1585. doi:10.1080/09546634.2023.2212059
13. Williams VL, Taylor SC, Onalaja AA. Scar management in racial/ethnic minorities: A systematic review of surgical approaches and outcomes. *Plast Reconstr Surg Glob Open.* 2024; **12**(1): e5578. doi:10.1097/GOX.0000000000005578
14. American Society for Dermatologic Surgery. 2023 ASDS Survey on dermatologic procedures. https://www.asds.net/medical-professionals/practice-resources/asds-survey-on-dermatologic-procedures. 2023.
15. Ziolkowski NI, Klassen AF, Mundy LR, *et al.* Cross-cultural validation of the SCAR-Q: Polish translation and international application. *Burns.* 2022; **48**(4): 922–930. doi:10.1016/j.burns.2021.08.023
16. Klassen AF, Ziolkowski N, Mundy LR, *et al.* SCAR-Q user's guide: Patient-reported outcomes instrument for individuals with scars. McMaster University. 2021. https://qportfolio.org/wp-content/uploads/2021/07/SCAR-Q-User-Guide_April-7-2021.pdf. Accessed April 12, 2024.

www.ingramcontent.com/pod-product-compliance
Lightning Source LLC
Chambersburg PA
CBHW081409061125
34979CB00006B/80
* 9 7 8 9 8 1 9 8 1 8 0 8 2 *